"This is an amazing book that will accelerate your journey to God-consciousness."

—**DEEPAK CHOPRA, author of *The Ultimate Happiness Prescription* and *Reinventing the Body, Resurrecting the Soul***

"This profound, beautiful, and pioneering book will ground the yoga community in a deeper mystical understanding, taking the worldwide yoga movement to a new level of inner empowerment and outer effectiveness. Whether you're a beginning student or a life-long practitioner, Andrew Harvey and Karuna Erickson will deepen your practice with this exalted and extremely practical book."

—**MARIANNE WILLIAMSON, author of *The Age of Miracles* and *The Healing of America***

"*Heart Yoga: The Sacred Marriage of Yoga and Mysticism* exquisitely merges the poetry of the Divine with the power of yoga with inspired precision. Authors Andrew Harvey and Karuna Erickson have accomplished the rigorous blending of heaven and earth, guaranteed to inspire new and well-seasoned students of yoga. This book is a magnificent accomplishment."

—**CAROLINE MYSS, author of *Entering the Castle* and *Anatomy of the Spirit***

"Andrew Harvey and Karuna Erickson have written an inspirational and passionate guide recognizing modern-day yogis as mystics on the mat. They invite us to experience our mats as temples, our movements as embodied prayer, the world as a divine altar, and our actions as the tools for change. *Heart Yoga* addresses how the awakening of the cosmic soul within the physical form inspires us to align our individual hearts with the universal call for action and service—the natural progression of yoga beyond the body. This is a magnificent and timely book affirming that the sacred practice of yoga is a journey of personal illumination, universal recognition, mystical unification, and the inevitable understanding that it is love and action that can transform this planet from one of fear and separation into one united by love, truth, and God."

—**SEANE CORN, yoga teacher, Global Yoga Ambassador for Youth AIDS, and co-visionary for "Off the Mat, Into the World"**

"*Heart Yoga: The Sacred Marriage of Yoga and Mysticism* is a potent offering with the depth of living wisdom, kindled knowledge, and mystical insight that will ignite the inherent fire of yoga lovers everywhere. The pages are infused with the direct passionate experience and wisdom of two longtime love pilgrims and scholars who are calling for and igniting the inner fire of the heart of yoga with piercing insight and a living joy. I have made Andrew Harvey's books a must-read in all our teacher trainings, and this is another sacred classic."

—SHIVA REA, founder and leading teacher of Prana Flow Yoga and Yoga Trance Dance™

"Karuna Erickson is delighting us with her authentic and intense inquiry into spirit. Her yoga is inspiring."

—RODNEY YEE, author of *Moving Toward Balance*

"Reading *Heart Yoga: The Sacred Marriage of Yoga and Mysticism* was a delicious revelation. Harvey and Erickson have blended the powerful practicality of yoga poses with the transcendent power of heart-opening spirituality in ways that are both inspiring and practicable for everyday life. I recommend it heartily to all students of yoga and self-transformation, as well as to those who simply want to live more deeply, more richly, and more happily."

—JUDITH HANSON LASATER, PhD, PT, yoga teacher since 1971 and author of *A Year of Living Your Yoga*

"As a longtime student and practitioner of yoga, I am filled with respect for *Heart Yoga: The Sacred Marriage of Yoga and Mysticism.* I particularly love this crystal-clear primer for practicing yoga as a means of connecting the body, mind, and spirit to all living beings. The frequent references to beautiful writings from all cultures and times make this book a rich and rewarding experience. I am inspired to take my own practice deeper, and to realize through it my own Sacred Activism, of which Andrew Harvey and Karuna Erickson have written so eloquently."

—ALI MCGRAW, actress

"This book is a quiet but passionate revelation. It takes the yoga community to a new level of process and empowerment. It invites all spiritual seekers to an adventure of embodiment. While being extremely ambitious and elevated, the book is also very lyrical, clear, and accessible. I believe that yoga is ready for the next wave and this book is it."

—DEBBIE FORD, author of *The Dark Side of the Light Chasers* and *Secret of the Shadows*

"Here is a wonderful gift to the world of today, a helpful Yoga container to develop fire in the heart, and beautiful meditations to inspire the heart's passion for the Great Work, both inner and the outer."

—PAUL H. RAY, coauthor of *The Cultural Creatives: How 50 Million People Are Changing the World*

"In *Heart Yoga,* Andrew Harvey and Karuna Erickson deliver an eloquent 'guidebook' to understanding and navigating the current evolution of yoga. This book strikes a fine balance between the transcendent powers of yoga, while providing understandable, practical, and effective techniques. Andrew and Karuna draw from vast experience, insight, and knowledge to provide a renewed sense of reverence to practitioners wishing to make their practice more sacred and inspired. *Heart Yoga* is perfectly timed to provide a tool to take one's practice and mystical inquiry to a new level of compassion, truth, and action in the world."

—ALLY BOGARD, Gaiatri Yoga, director of yoga teacher training and international yoga teacher

"We are delighted to see this beautiful book that ... reveals what so many of us have long known—that the real work of life is to open ourselves to living in our spiritual heart center. This book provides both practical and spiritual guidance as you move forward on your journey into Self! Bravo, Karuna and Andrew!"

—NICKI DOANE and EDDIE MODESTINI, Maya Yoga Studio, Maui, Hawaii

ALSO BY ANDREW HARVEY

The Hope: A Guide to Sacred Activism

A Walk with Four Spiritual Guides: Krishna, Buddha, Jesus, and Ramakrishna

The Way of Passion

The Return of the Mother

The Essential Mystics: Selections from the World's Great Wisdom Traditions

Love's Glory: Re-creations of Rumi

Light Upon Light: Inspirations from Rumi

A Journey in Ladakh: Encounters with Buddhism

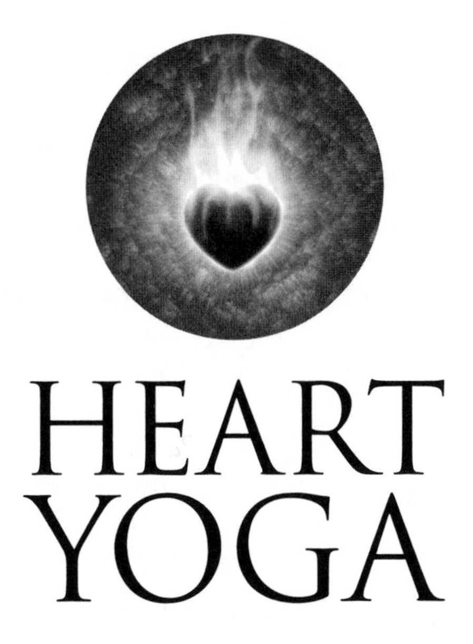

HEART YOGA

THE SACRED MARRIAGE OF YOGA AND MYSTICISM

ANDREW HARVEY & KARUNA ERICKSON

North Atlantic Books
Berkeley, California

Published by
North Atlantic Books
P.O. Box 12327
Berkeley, California 94712

Cover art ©istockphoto.com/stereohype
Cover and book design by Suzanne Albertson
Photographs by Ricardo Hubbs

Printed in the United States of America

NOTE: Every effort has been made to locate the artist in order to acquire permission to reprint an element that appears on the cover. Please contact North Atlantic Books if you are the artist or have information on how to locate them.

Heart Yoga: The Sacred Marriage of Yoga and Mysticism is sponsored by the Society for the Study of Native Arts and Sciences, a nonprofit educational corporation whose goals are to develop an educational and cross-cultural perspective linking various scientific, social, and artistic fields; to nurture a holistic view of arts, sciences, humanities, and healing; and to publish and distribute literature on the relationship of mind, body, and nature.

North Atlantic Books' publications are available through most bookstores. For further information, visit our Web site at www.northatlanticbooks.com or call 800-733-3000.

Library of Congress Cataloging-in-Publication Data

Harvey, Andrew, 1952–
Heart yoga : the sacred marriage of yoga and mysticism / Andrew Harvey and Karuna Erickson.
p. cm.
Summary: "Illustrated by beautiful photographs and quotations from the world's spiritual traditions, Heart Yoga presents the practice of hatha yoga as a spiritual path leading to mystical union with the divine"—Provided by publisher.
Includes bibliographical references.
ISBN 978-1-55643-897-4
1. Hatha yoga. 2. Mysticism. I. Erickson, Karuna. II. Title.
BL1238.56.H38H37 2010
204'.36—dc22

2010001952

1 2 3 4 5 6 7 8 9 SHERIDAN 15 14 13 12 11 10

To my beloved life-partner Paul, and to our inspiring children Amanda, Eli, and Mosang, with deep gratitude for your infinite kindness, compassion, wisdom, patience, and faith in me, as well as to my grandson and grandmother—my teachers of joy and delight.

—Karuna

To my beloved friend Ali McGraw, for her passion, irreverence, courage, loyalty, loving defense of animal rights, and pioneering love of yoga.

—Andrew

To the great yogis and mystics of all the traditions, who have given their lives to birthing the divine in the human and to embodying the fire of the Sacred Heart in Sacred Activism. May any merit that comes to us from this book be offered to the healing and illumination of all beings. May all those who come to Heart Yoga experience and celebrate the love that is the inherent quality of their heart.

—Karuna and Andrew

The Spirit shall look out through Matter's gaze
And Matter shall reveal the Spirit's face
And all the Earth become a single life.

—SRI AUROBINDO

CONTENTS

Foreword by Rodney Yee

Several years ago I was sitting with Andrew Harvey and Karuna Erickson in a cozy hotel lobby in downtown Oakland. I was pondering the project that might spring forth from our provocative meeting. Karuna had been the catalyst for this gathering and was radiating enthusiasm for the possibilities. What she did not realize then was that I was an unnecessary part to the puzzle.

I knew that Karuna had received all that I had to offer as her teacher, and that she was ripe to deliver so many crucial messages in her own voice. She had become so nuanced in her understanding of yoga, and was adding a necessary feminine awakening to the evolution. As we talked over tea and cakes, I was spellbound by Andrew Harvey and his poetic description of the evolution of consciousness and the next step in our journey together. Almost in a state of divine play and dialogue, he held space for the three of us to share.

Many signs are appearing that are telling us about a great shift that is going to occur. There is going to be a quantum leap, jumping from an old paradigm to a completely new understanding. There are necessary techniques and preparations that we must practice to make this transition peacefully and consciously. Andrew and Karuna have written one of the essential manuals that takes us step by step through this threshold.

The rest is in your hands; read the manual and then practice, practice, practice. Like Andrew and Karuna, you must embody the teachings and make them your own. Through their inspiration and guidance we can begin the inner journey that will inspire us to be free from the shackles of today's unhealthy perspective of isolation and separateness. When we see others as ourselves and break the old perception of who we think we are, we can return to wholeness and heal the wounds that have manifested from our myopic vision.

I thank my friends for this wonderful offering that has arisen from countless hours of work and play, and their lifetimes of devoted practice.

—Rodney Yee

Introduction

Body must be made spirit for spirit to become body.

—attributed to HERMES TRISMEGISTUS, the priest who introduced the art of alchemy to Egypt, 2500 BCE

I am practicing asana but at a level where the quality is meditative. The totality of being, from core to skin, is experienced. Mind is unruffled, intelligence is awake in heart rather than in head, self is quiescent, and conscious life is in every cell of the body. That is what I mean when I say asana opens up the whole spectrum of yoga's possibilities.

—B. K. S. IYENGAR[1]

The masters say that the Great Work consists in corporealizing the spirit and spiritualizing the body, in making fluid the fixed, the body, in fixing and stabilizing the fluid, the spirit, in manifesting the Mystery and in making mysterious the manifest. The philosopher's stone, the final product of alchemy, is the spirit arrived at the density and concrete reality of a body . . . I raise myself to God to compel Him to descend into my being and to give birth to Him. And for that I must have a body, a belly; my body must exist in my soul; I must develop a strong body, powerful, sensual, sexual, volcanic, fertile . . . Oh, I love life!

—ETIENNE PERROT, *The Way of Transformation*

Fuse the powers of the sacred heart with the energies of the body, and you can transform everything.

—PIERRE TEILHARD DE CHARDIN

Heart Yoga is the marriage of the yoga of the illumined body with the mysticism of the awakened heart. The time has come to restore this ancient marriage to its full power. Heart Yoga offers, at these chaotic and difficult times, the union of grounded passion and peaceful joy in the core of the body and heart that everyone needs to keep strong, creative, and inspired by love. As Rumi wrote, "Are all the candles out? Hand them to a lover ... A lover's soul stays fresh, vibrant, light."[2] Heart Yoga brings to all those who practice it with devotion this fresh, light vibrancy of being.

Nothing is more important for us now than to root our whole beings in the heart-fire energies of the dance of the universe. Mystics of every tradition have experienced these calm, tender, and luminous energies. They have recognized them both as the birthing powers of reality and as fountains of continual renewal flowing perpetually from the heart of the One Heart.

Yoga was created by the ancient sages of India to be a healing and transforming gift for the entire world. It was intended to help everybody become embodied channels of illumined love, grace, and peace, and so, instruments of divine creativity and service in the world. In their forest hermitages, these yogis were inspired by a vision of the unity of all reality, of the Sacred Marriage between matter and light, earth and heaven, body and spirit, awakened heart and mind. As the Dalai Lama has written, matter and mind are but "different aspects of an indivisible reality," and "matter in its subtlest form is *prana,* a vital energy which is inseparable from consciousness ... Because of this indivisibility of consciousness and energy, there is a profoundly intimate correlation between the elements within our bodies and the natural elements in the outside world. This subtle connection can be discerned by individuals who have gained a certain level of spiritual realization or who have a naturally higher level of perception."[3]

The ancient yogis were such individuals. They evolved postures and meditations that could gently guide others into the compassionate oneness with all things and the celebratory joy that they experienced to be the essence of reality. Yoga essentially is a way of joyfully offering thanks, and of honoring the Divine presence in all of creation. The wisdom of the creators of yoga is simply and profoundly expressed in a timeless yogic text:

> From joy all beings have come.
> In joy all beings are sustained.
> To joy all beings return.
> This is the highest teaching.
> This is the highest teaching.
> —UPANISHADS

These sages merged their yoga practice with mystical meditation, bringing body and soul into unity. In this union, the whole being fills with radiant health, and glows in the joy that creates and sustains all things.

When yoga is practiced with conscious knowledge of its vast original purpose, and in union with simple, luminous, and profound meditations, it awakens this joyful praise of existence in every cell of the body. It gives those who practice it with devotion increasing access to an inexhaustible well of divine energy. With grace, it gradually initiates practitioners into that experience of celebration mystics have described as the essence of life. As it is said in the Upanishads: "The wise see Love flaming in all creation, and their hearts are filled with wonder."

Heart Yoga offers to everybody, and to every body, a direct path into this vision of Love flaming in all creation, and the wonder and radical self-empowerment that flows from it. This empowerment fuels us to act with a lucid and sacred passion in the world. We believe that the way forward now for the human race lies in what we call Sacred Activism. Sacred Activism is the marriage in every part of one's being, between the fire of the mystic's passion for God and the fire of the activist's passion for justice. This marriage of these powerful spiritual fires engenders a third fire, the heart-fire of love in action. This is an intense, all-transformative energy that provides the fuel for a quantum leap in human evolution. Heart Yoga is a crucible that can calmly and fully birth this third fire. Heart Yoga grounds this fire in the peace, strength, and stamina which will allow it to go on burning, whatever the challenges and demands.

The profound meaning and precious gift of yoga is its source in the unity of body and spirit. Yoga's great inspiration is that it expresses, in both philosophy and practice, the Sacred Marriage of transcendence and immanence, heaven and earth, masculine and feminine, spirit and body. All the seeming dualities unite as One, and are experienced as One, always One. Rumi writes of this experience,

> Define and narrow me, you starve yourself of yourself.
> Nail me down in a box of cold words, that box is your coffin.
> I do not know who I am.
> I am in astounding lucid confusion.
> I am not a Christian, I am not a Jew, I am not a Zoroastrian,
> And I am not even a Muslim.
> I do not belong to the land, or to any known or unknown sea.
> Nature cannot own or claim me, nor can heaven,
> Nor can India,
> China, Bulgaria,
> My birthplace is placelessness,
> My sign to have and give no sign.
> You say you see my mouth, ears, eyes, nose—they are not mine.
> I am the life of life.
> I am that cat, this stone, no one.
> I have thrown duality away like an old dishrag,
> I see and know all times and worlds,
> As one, one, always one.
> So what do I have to do to get you to admit who is speaking?
> Admit it and change everything!
> This is your own voice echoing off the walls of God.[4]

Over the past decade there has been a tremendous resurgence of interest in yoga. Millions of yoga students all over the world have experienced the profound benefits of yoga practice. Often the emphasis of their practice has been on the physical aspects of yoga, which are the most easily communicated, and are of course extraordinarily beneficial. One potential shadow of this concentration on the physical aspects of yoga is to limit the vision of the vast transformative potential of yoga, and a tendency to self-absorption. We believe that this shadow needs now to be seen and compassionately healed by restoring to our modern yoga practice its ancient and liberating mystical depths. At this time in our history, we need the ancient practices and wisdom of yoga to sustain, inspire, and encourage us to respond in healing ways to the many world crises. The subtle depth of the vision of yoga needs to be recaptured and expressed in its full power.

This is why, after decades of study and practice, we offer this book, *Heart Yoga*. We all are now called to be on fire with both divine passion and divine peace, glowing with inner heart-fire to meet the challenges of our burning world, fueled by sacred energy to act to preserve our planet. This book presents the vision and practices that will ignite and fan the divine spark we each carry into a heart bonfire. This bonfire, burning in every cell of our hearts, minds, souls and bodies, will give us the energy and vision to heal and transform our planet. The Buddha, in his Fire Sermon, spoke of a humanity burning tragically in the fires of anger, ignorance, greed, and delusion. It is our experience that Heart Yoga engenders a fire that meets these fires and transmutes them. This transmutation contains the key to the future of humanity, and is the alchemy that can birth the divine in the human.

May all beings drink deeply of Heart Yoga's cup of sacred celebration. May all beings unite illumined body and awakened heart in love for and service to all sentient beings in our burning world. As Teilhard de Chardin wrote,

> Love
> is the free and imaginative outflowing
> of the Spirit over all unexplored paths.

It links those
who love in bonds that unite,
but do not destroy, causing them to discover in their mutual contact
an exaltation capable of stirring in the very core
of their being all that they possess
of uniqueness and creative power.
Love alone
can unite living beings
so as to complete and fulfill them,
for it alone joins them by what is deepest
in themselves. All we need
is to imagine our ability to love
developing until it embraces the totality
of the people of the Earth.
Theoretically
this transformation of love is quite possible.
What paralyzes life is failure to believe
and failure to dare.
The day will come when,
After harnessing space,
the winds,
the tides,
and gravitation,
We shall harness for God the energies of love.
And on that day, for the second time
in the history of the world,
We shall have discovered fire.[5]

OM SHANTI SHANTI SHANTI

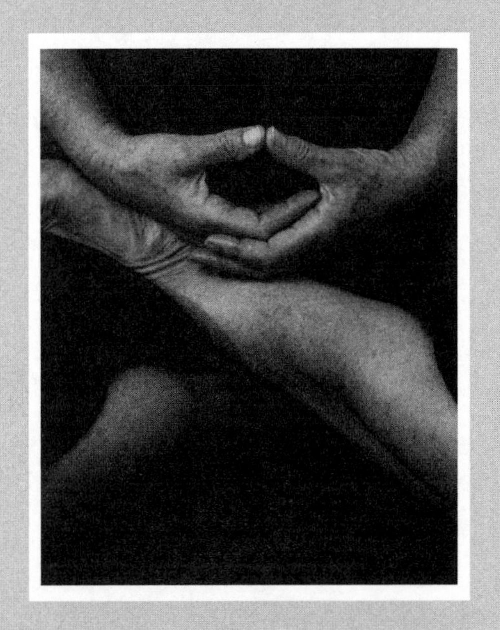

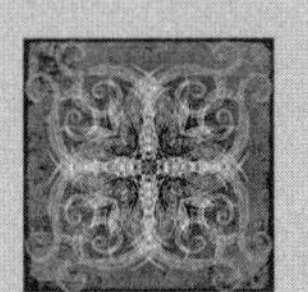 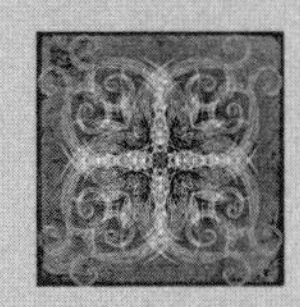 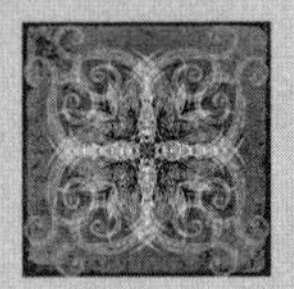

ONE

Preparing for the Practice of Heart Yoga

Devotion

It is only through devotion and devotion alone, that you will realize the absolute truth.

—THE BUDDHA

Practice

The Blessed Goddess said:

"Whenever one does anything, one has no success whatsoever without practice *(abhyasa).*"

The sages know this to be practice: being dedicated to one thing, reflecting upon it, talking about it with one another, and understanding it.

—YOGA-VASISHTHA[1]

Mystics of the Marriage: The Journey of the Soul

The purpose of the soul entering this body is to display her powers and actions in this world, for she needs an instrument. By descending to this world, she increases the flow of her power to guide the human being through the world. Thereby she perfects herself above and below, attaining a higher state by being fulfilled in all dimensions. If she is not fulfilled both above and below, she is not complete.

Before descending to this world, the soul is emanated from the mystery of the highest level. While in this world, she is completed and fulfilled by this lower world. Departing this world, she is filled with the fullness of all the worlds, the world above and the world below.

At first, before descending to this world, the soul is imperfect; she is lacking something. By descending to this world, she is perfected in every dimension.

—MOSES DE LEON[2]

The New Body

> The body will be turned by the power of the spiritual consciousness into a true and fit and perfectly responsive instrument of the Spirit. This new relation of the spirit and the body assumes—and makes possible—a free acceptance of the whole of material Nature ... As a result of this new relation between the Spirit and the body, the Gnostic evolution will effectuate the spiritualization, perfection and fulfillment of the physical being.
>
> —SRI AUROBINDO[3]

Preparing the whole being for Heart Yoga means opening up your entire self—heart, mind, soul, and body—to the vision and experience of the Sacred Marriage. The Sacred Marriage is the dynamic and endlessly fertile dance of seeming dualities that are secretly interconnected: transcendence and immanence, absolute and relative reality, light and matter, masculine and feminine, mind and heart, soul and body. It is this ecstatic dance, the mystics of all traditions tell us, that is ceaselessly birthing the universes and appearing as them in every cell of the body. As the Hindu mystic Jnaneshwar wrote:

> Without the God
> There is no Goddess,
> And without the Goddess
> There is no God.
> How sweet is their love!
> The entire universe
> is too small to contain them,
> Yet they live happily
> in the tiniest particle.[4]

In the vision of the Sacred Marriage, we begin to see with joy, wonder, and reverence that the whole meaning of us being here is to experience this sacred dance of God and Goddess in the tiniest particles of our bodies, and for our bodies to be transformed ever more deeply into light-matter. We are here to embody the transcendent.

In the Bible it is written (I Corinthians:6–19) that our bodies are the temples of the Holy Spirit, which is within us. In the Koran, God describes the act of the creation of humanity as "I breathe into him, Adam, my spirit" (Sura 28, verse 72). The body is, in other words, the living locus of the presence of the Spirit. By virtue of that presence, in the tiniest particle, the body is the most holy of temples. It was this recognition that flowered in the sacred architecture of Egypt, ancient India and Asia, and medieval Europe. The great temples and cathedrals are all conscious embodiments of the divine human.

These temples are architecturally constructed to represent the exact proportions of the human body. The buildings themselves are manifestations of the Sacred Marriage between spirit and body that gives birth to the divine child. Knowing this, when you enter these houses of the divine, you will experience your own body as the house of divine light-consciousness and love. These temples transmit the experience of the reality of the body's great task of embodying the living presence of the Divine. This great work of embodiment births in every part of us a divine force of passionate compassion. We become embodied flames of the great fire of the Sacred Marriage, which is at all times burning in reality.

In Southern India in Chidambaram, at the holiest of all the temples to the dancing Shiva, the Lord of the Universe is worshipped as the Golden Dancer. Every morning a golden image of Shiva is brought out to the chanting of ancient Sanskrit hymns, so that the universe can be recreated in the splendor of his living presence. Heart Yoga, the yoga of the Sacred Marriage, enables you to experience your radical union with the golden dancer, and to allow yourself, through practice, to become one with the dance. You unite in the very depths of your cells with that divine light-consciousness, that bliss of compassion that, as Dante says, "moves the sun and the stars," and you discover for yourself with humble awe and grateful rapture the all-transforming truth that is enshrined in the ninth-century Buddhist monk-poet Saraha's words:

> Here in the body are the sacred rivers Jamuna and Ganges. Here are Prashna and Benares, the Sun and the Moon. In my wanderings I have visited many sanctuaries, but none more holy than that of my body.[5]

Since, as we have seen, the body is the most sacred of sanctuaries, when we begin practice we need to create a sacred space in which we can experience our own divine identity, just as in the world's great places of worship. This is far less challenging than it may sound; in fact, the greater the simplicity of devotion with which you approach this task, the more powerful your experience of union will be. The divine presence is, as the medieval alchemists said, the "absolutely simple thing." The simpler and more one-pointed our devotion to the divine, the more profoundly the divine's own radiance can appear to us, in us, as us. As Kabir reminds us,

> Only while you are alive is there hope of finding him. . . .
> It is a hopeless dream
> To think that union will come after the soul leaves the body.
> What you get now
> is what you get then. . . .
> Kabir says, "Only spiritual practice will get you across;
> be addicted to this practice."[6]

Creating a Sacred Space

In a time like ours, the creation of sacred space is not only an act of celebration of the Sacred Marriage, it is an urgent prayer for sacred order. Knowing and feeling this will lend your practice, from the beginning, a heightened calm intensity and clarity. It will help you remember that the true aim of Heart Yoga is not only your own transformation, but the transformation of all the unjust and oppressive conditions of the world that create suffering. In other words, allowing yourself to be penetrated by the full significance of what it means to invoke and create sacred space will help you dedicate your journey in Heart Yoga to the happiness and liberation, not only of yourself, but all sentient beings. It will give you a way of responding directly to the deepest needs of our times, as well as a way of meeting those needs without stress, in a state of surrendered joy. To enter this urgent yet calm, focused yet surrendered, intention for your practice, let this extraordinary message from the Hopi elders speak to every cell of your being.

Message from the Hopi Elders

We have been telling the people that this is the Eleventh Hour
Now you must go back and tell the people that this is the Hour
And there are things to be considered.
Where are you living?
What are you doing?
What are your relationships?
Are you in right relation?
Where is your water?
Know your garden.
It is time to speak your truth
Create your community.
Be good to each other.
And do not look outside yourself for the leader.
This could be a good time!
There is a river flowing now very fast
It is so great and swift that there are those who will be afraid.
They will try to hold on to the shore.
They will feel they are being torn apart and they will suffer greatly.
Know the river has its destination.

The elders say we must let go of the shore, and push off into the river,
Keep our eyes open, and our heads above water.
See who is in there with you and celebrate.
At this time in history, we are to take nothing personally,
least of all ourselves.
For the moment that we do,
our spiritual growth and journey comes to a halt.
The time of the lone wolf is over. Gather yourselves!
Banish the word "struggle" from your attitude and your vocabulary.
All that you do now must be done in a sacred manner and in celebration.
We are the ones we have been waiting for. . . .

—THE ELDERS, Hopi Nation, Oraibi, Arizona, June 8, 2000

Setting Intention: Beginning in a Sacred Way

All that you do now, as the Hopi elders remind us, must be done in a sacred way, and in celebration. This is especially true of selecting and creating the space in which you are going to experience your body as a temple, which is going to be the radiant, alchemical crucible of your embodiment of the light, your own transformation into the golden dancer.

Select a place in your home that is as quiet as possible. You may wish to create an altar on which you could place any symbols that inspire you and call you to the essence of your vision of your deepest self and of the fully embodied divine human you long to realize. The creation of an altar to inspire and dedicate your practice is a very personal act. You might bring together on your altar images of the divine, pictures of teachers or friends you love, flowers, candles, special stones—anything that deeply speaks to you of illumination, inspiration, and sacred presence. On Andrew's altar are images of the God and Goddess in ecstatic union, photos of dear friends, pictures of Mary and the Christ, stones from all over the world, and an old Mexican good luck charm. On Karuna's altar are candles, sage for burning, photos of ancestors and children, flowers, sacred carvings, and special gifts from heart friends. Tending to our altars and meditating on the objects on them over time gives our altars extraordinary power to infuse us with divine presence. On the occasion of Karuna's sixtieth birthday, her heart friends built a beautiful altar for her in the center of her home, and placed carefully created or chosen gifts upon it to inspire and guide her practice and to bless her journey with their love, embodied in these symbols.

When you begin your practice, make sure you enter completely into the present moment. In silence, tune into the voice of your heart and allow it to form an intention or prayer that will guide your practice. You may want to dedicate your practice to the liberation of all sentient beings, or stream the merits of your practice toward the welfare of a being in need. Whatever focus you choose or prayer you make, make it consciously and deeply, so that all your ensuing practice will unfold from this sacred place. One suggested prayer to use is from the Buddhist tradition: "May from the merits of my practice all sentient beings everywhere be liberated from all suffering." Another possibility is repeating the first line of the great prayer of St Francis: "Lord, make me an instrument of thy peace."

At first you might not be clear about your intention for this practice. Just let go and trust that inspiration will come. As Rumi wrote, "For sixty years I have been forgetful every moment, but not for a second has this flowing toward me stopped or slowed."[7] Sit or lie on your mat for a while, immersed in this flowing, and relaxing and listening to your body and mind. The place of not-knowing is rich and fertile. In beginner's mind you are open to everything. Wait until an intention emerges that resonates throughout your body, mind, and heart. You can trust your intuition to guide you into the heart of your own authentic practice.

It is important to set a conscious intention to give yourself an uninterrupted time for practice, so that the outer distractions of daily living won't disturb your immersion in devotion. Choose not to follow compulsions to do something else that suddenly looks crucial, like answering the phone, email, laundry, or dishes! For some people, practicing at the same time each day for a specific time period helps them stay disciplined. Others, especially parents of young children, just practice whenever they can! Whatever your current circumstances, make sure you honor your true self by giving yourself some time each day to savor its presence.

Gather Your Supplies

All you really "need" is a yoga mat so that your feet won't slip in standing poses. It's easy to buy one online or at a yoga studio, but if you don't have one, you can still practice on the floor or a thin carpet. You might also enjoy using props like blankets, blocks, straps, bolsters, a chair, or an eye pillow. These props support you in easing into the poses more gently. Never force your body into a pose, but instead use these props to adapt the pose to suit the needs of your own unique body. In India there are holy days in which workers bless the tools of their trade and recognize them as precious gifts of the divine. Healers of different traditions bless and keep sacred their instruments to honor, thank, and keep them charged with divine powers. Objects used in sacred ceremonies all over the world are always maintained in a way that symbolizes their holy and precious nature. What ceremony could be more sacred than experiencing and uniting with your truest essence? Your yoga mat, props, meditation shawl, etc., are not only useful objects, they are holy. As you continue your practice, they become more charged with the power of your practice. Keep them in their own safe place and treat them with reverence and gratitude.

Consult a Health Professional

Heart Yoga is designed to be practically attuned to the needs of each unique individual. The energies it opens up in you can be powerfully healing, but you must always listen to the wisdom of your own body. As Seyyed Hossein Nasr so beautifully expresses, "The body, in fact, has its own intelligence and speaks its own 'mind,' reflecting a wisdom before which the response of any human intelligence not dulled by pseudo-knowledge or veiled by pride and the passions can only be wonder and awe at the Wisdom of the Creator."[8]

Most of the poses we suggest in this book are quite basic and can be adapted for every body. However, there are various contraindications to practicing some poses. Please consult with a qualified health professional or experienced yoga teacher before beginning practice, especially if you have any medical condition requiring treatment, if you are recovering from an injury, illness, or surgery, or if you have any of the following conditions: pregnancy; joint or spinal disk injury; hypertension; glaucoma; back, neck, or shoulder problems; hernia; sciatica; retinal problems; heart problems; or any other medical concerns. Heart Yoga can be healing and therapeutic for many of these conditions if the practice is done with skillful guidance and awareness.

Preparing the Heart for Heart Yoga

Now we have come to the moment of beginning the practice of Heart Yoga. Patanjali begins his Yoga Sutras (I-1) with the Sanskrit words *"Atha Yoganushasanam,"* which translates, "Now, at this auspicious moment of transition, begins our study of the practice of yoga according to the ancient tradition."[9] At this sacred beginning, it is essential that all practitioners of Heart Yoga truly understand what is meant by the heart. The heart in yogic and mystical terms is not the actual physical heart. Heart Yoga, while being suffused with sacred emotion, must never be confused with a yoga of emotions. What we mean by the heart is the heart center of the psycho-spiritual body, in which, as all mystical traditions know, the physical body is contained—and by which it is illumined.

This heart center is known in all mystical traditions. In Hinduism it is called the *anahata*. In Sufi mysticism it is known as the center of the royal king. In Christian mysticism it is called the Sacred Heart. Its presence is felt, when it is awakened, an inch or two to the right of the middle of the chest.

When it is open, it pulses gently with a sweet intense fire that is the direct experience of in-dwelling love.

The heart center is especially sacred to the mystics of the Sacred Marriage because they know it to be the placeless place in which the God and the Goddess, transcendence and immanence, make incessant and ecstatic love. It is, in other words, the marriage bed of the Mother-Father, the bed of divine light in which they experience each other's radiance and bliss.

The heart center is the clue to the transforming power of Heart Yoga. Just as the physical heart pumps blood around the physical body to keep it fresh, vibrant, and alive, so, when through devotion and mystical experience the heart center is opened, it circulates the fire, energy, and light power of the Mother-Father, both in the psycho-spiritual and the physical body.

This supreme secret of the transformation of the entire being has been known in the esoteric traditions. The great orthodox Christian mystic of the fourth century, St. Makarios, describes this "heart."

> The heart governs and reigns over the whole bodily organism . . . and when grace possesses the ranges of the heart, it rules over all the members and the thoughts. For there in the heart is the mind, and all the thoughts of the soul and its expectations, and in this way grace penetrates also to all the members of the body.[10]

Seyyed Hossein Nasr, our greatest contemporary Islamic spiritual philosopher, describes the Sufi vision of this heart center in an essay on Islamic mysticism, *The Throne of the All-Merciful,* that

> . . . the heart is the center of the human microcosm . . . the meeting place between the human and the celestial realms where the spirit resides, the isthmus between this world and the next, between the visible and invisible worlds, between the human realm and the realm of the spirit, between the horizontal and vertical dimensions of existence . . . how remarkable is this reality of the heart, that mysterious center which from the point of view of our earthly

> experience seems so small, and yet, as the Prophet has said, it is the Throne [*Al-Arsh*] of God the All-Merciful [*Al-Rahman*], the Throne that encompasses the whole universe.[11]

The ancient sages of India who created yoga tell us in the Chandogya Upanishad:

> As great as the infinite space beyond is the space within the lotus of the heart. Both heaven and earth are contained in that inner space, both fire and air, sun and moon, lightning and stars. Whether we know it in this world or know it not, everything is contained in that inner space.[12]

May these three sublime evocations of the power and glory of the heart center inspire you as you begin your practice. May you enter into devoted relation with this divine reality within you, through which all the energies of the Mother-Father can flow, to transform you in heart, mind, soul, and body.

The mystical traditions that honor the transforming primacy of the heart center know that there is one very simple way of invoking its presence. This is by repeating the name of God, or a mantra or short prayer that profoundly moves you. In Sufi mysticism this is called polishing the heart.

A great ninth-century Sufi mystic, Najm al-Din Kubra, describes precisely the unfolding of the sacred technology of transfiguration that is initiated by the recitation of the name or prayer or mantra.

> There are lights which ascend and lights which descend. The ascending lights are the lights of the heart; the descending lights are those of the Throne [the transcendent Godhead]. The false self is the veil between the Throne and the heart. When this veil is torn, and a door opens in the heart, like springs toward like. Light ascends toward light and light descends upon light, and it is "light upon light." [Koran 24:35]
>
> When each time the heart sighs for the throne the throne sighs for the heart, so they come to meet. Each time a light ascends from you, a light

> descends toward you. If their energies are equal, then they meet halfway. But when the substance of light has grown in you, then this makes up a whole in relation to what is in the same nature in Heaven. Then, it is the substance of light in Heaven that longs for you, and is drawn to your light, and it descends toward you. This is the secret of the mystical journey.[13]

What this description of transfiguration reveals is the core, essence, and power of Heart Yoga. When through calm meditation and passionate devotion the heart center is completely opened and the lover has become the beloved of the Beloved, the eternal light of the Beloved then pours ceaselessly down from the crown center into the heart center to illumine the mind, irradiate and divinize all emotions, awakening all the cells of the body to their blissful light-nature.

We suggest that before you begin your physical practice you prepare the invisible sacred crucible in which that practice will take place. Say a name of the Divine that you love, choose a mantra, or use a line of a prayer such as "Lord, make me an instrument of Thy peace." One beautiful way of invoking the presence of the heart is to sit cross-legged and bow your head slightly toward your heart, with your hands folded over your heart in prayer. Bowing the head to the heart is recommended in the Christian, Sufi, Hindu, and Buddhist traditions as a most direct and powerful way of reminding yourself that your mind and its reason are made whole by being the servants of the luminous intelligence of the heart. We recommend one particular mantra, for those who love to practice yoga within the sacred atmosphere of the tradition that created it. This mantra is known as the Gayatri Mantra. In the Bhagavad Gita, Krishna says, "Of meters I am the Gayatri." In the chapter, "Meditation on the Gayatri," the Chandogya Upanishad states, "The Gayatri is everything, whatever here exists. Speech is verily the Gayatri, for speech sings forth [*gaya-ti*] and protects [*traya-te*] whatever here exists." The Chandogya Upanishad also tells us that "Gayatri is also the earth, for everything that exists here rests on this earth and does not go beyond. In man, that Gayatri is also the body, for the pranas exist in this body and do not go beyond. That body, in man is again the heart within a man; for the pranas exist in it and do not go beyond."[14]

Swami Adiswarananda, in his definitive work *Meditation and Its Practices,* says of the Gayatri Mantra:

> The Gayatri Mantra is the essence of all mantras . . . it embodies in itself mystically all the meters and all the seers of all other mantras and their presiding deities, as well as the glory of those deities. By invoking the Gayatri all these are invoked in oneself. By the repetition of this mantra, every sacred mantra is repeated.[15]

The Gayatri Mantra is found in the most ancient Indian scriptures, the Rig Veda. In Sanskrit it reads as follows:

> OM BHUR BHUVAH SWAH;
> TAT SAVITUR-VARENYAM
> BHARGO DEVASYA DHIMAHI;
> DHIYO YO NAH PRACHODAYAT. OM.

Father Bede Griffiths, Andrew's beloved teacher, once translated the Gayatri Mantra for him in this way: "We meditate on the radiance of the Divine Light. May that Divine Light lead us to the realization of the Truth." Swami Adiswarananda offers these beautiful instructions when repeating the mantra:

> When meditating on the Gayatri mantra, the seeker is instructed to direct his attention to the radiant light of the sun. From this he is led to meditate on the source of the light of perception and understanding within, without which one cannot perceive the light of the sun. In the final stage, he is asked to meditate on the identity of the light in him and the light of the sun—the identity of the Pure Consciousness of his inner Self and the all-pervading Pure Consciousness of the universal Self.[16]

One powerful way, then, that you can realize the presence of the heart is to visualize it as a sun pulsing and radiating in the core of your chest. Visualize that sun strongly, allowing its rays to penetrate every cell of your body and to create a field spreading out about six feet beyond and around your body. The sun within is now the sun-field of the radiant heart in which your practice will unfold.

Dedication of Your Practice

After preparing the heart, it is essential in Heart Yoga to let the heart's unconditional love for all beings express itself in a dedication of all the merits of your practice to the liberation of all sentient beings everywhere from suffering and to the transformation of the world. We offer the following prayer that we use, and invite you to create one that expresses your own deepest longing for yourself and the world. "May all benefits flowing to me through this practice of Heart Yoga be freely offered as a prayer for the liberation of all sentient beings. May all beings be filled with peace, love, and joy."

Practical Hints for Heart Yoga

Your practice is a prayer, your expression of honoring your own life and honoring life itself. People often wonder how to choose their own practice each day. The answer is simple: become the alchemist of your own transformation by choosing whatever practice you need to bring balance to your present situation. When you sense you need to wake yourself up, choose an active, energetic practice. When you need to relax, a peaceful, restorative practice is best. Sometimes a balanced sequence of both energetic and peaceful poses is beneficial. Observe where your body and mind are drawn, experimenting with letting go of any plan or agenda about what you should do, and responding to what feels right in the moment.

At times a focused practice, directly related to your current physical or emotional state, is appropriate. If you feel stuck in crisis or obsessed with a problem, for example, choose an expansive, spacious practice like the Joy of Transcendence practice. When you feel dissociated or blank, return to an earthy harmony and feel your kinship with all life with a grounded practice like the Joy of Creation practice. If you feel withdrawn, lonely, or depressed, choose a practice that releases the heart energy such as the Joy of Love of all Beings practice. When you feel separate, you can focus on renewing your connection with yourself or another with a practice emphasizing relationship like the Joy of Tantra. When you want to feel encouragement or passion to act in the world, choose a practice that awakens you to the Joy of Service. Explore an energizing practice to inspire strength and courage when you feel lethargic or afraid. A restorative practice helps you to relax deeply, restore your energy, and move beyond your ego to your vibrant connection with all beings and to your heart's natural inclination to care for others.

Some days you'll be feeling joyful, peaceful, or in a state of expansive well-being, and you'll choose a practice that naturally emerges from, expresses, and enhances that state. Over time you'll naturally move toward a practice that arises authentically from your deepest essence.

Whatever practice you choose, don't let yoga become yet another part of your "self-improvement program" where you're trying to change who you are and get "better."

Let gentleness be your guide. The essence of gentleness is its fusion of yielding and strength, which is the source of its power to harmonize and heal. *Ahimsa,* or non-harming, is the essential root and foundation of all yoga practice, because practicing in its spirit fills the body with the tenderness of Divine Love. B. K. S. Iyengar explains that *ahimsa* "is more than a negative command . . . it has a wider positive meaning, love."[17] As we relate to the body, so we relate to the world. A body at peace with itself radiates the peace of compassion to others.

Rooted in this compassion, let your practice be a way to observe deeply and respond skillfully to how you're feeling. Practice simply for the love of the practice, just because it feels true for you. This creates a spaciousness in your practice and in your being that is essential for healing and transformation.

Your mind or will alone will not help you choose which practice is best for you. Listen and be guided by your inner wisdom. Beginners may wish to stay with the suggested sequences in this book for a while. More experienced students will add poses to lengthen and deepen their practice. After a while, you'll learn to trust your intuition, your own inner teacher, and explore your own natural sequences of movement. Be curious, explore your inner experience, and let it evolve.

Trust yourself to sense when to move into and out of poses. There is no prescribed time to stay in each pose. In general, at least five breaths will give you time to align your body and explore how you're feeling, but in many poses you'll want to stay longer.

Never push or force yourself into any position. The foundation of yoga rests in non-violence *(ahimsa)* and truth *(satya)*. Honor yourself by being fully present with compassion and joy, and this will prepare you to enter the deep meditative and transformative states that the practices are designed to engender. Compassion is the beginning, the means, and the end of Heart Yoga, because it is through compassion that we are most seamlessly connected to the infinite energy of the universe.

Recently Karuna was blessed to attend a yoga class in Costa Rica taught by a radiant seventy-nine-year-old woman, who looked to be in her forties and has practiced yoga since the 1950s. It was extraordinary how long she could hold the poses. Karuna sat at her feet afterwards and asked, "Tell me about your practice of sixty years." She simply replied, "Well, you know, there's infinite energy in the universe. And yoga is about connecting with this infinite energy." Her practice was beautiful, because she was both so absorbed and awake in it, and naturally compassionate with herself. She exemplified the deep truth of yoga, that yoga is an inner marriage of the body with the Infinite Beloved, and that what is essential is not physical perfection, but authentic inner abandon to Spirit. As Patanjali expressed, "Asana is mastered when there is relaxation and meditation on the Infinite." (Yoga Sutras, II-47) From this meditation, a fountain of bliss-energy flows.

Resistance

It is easy to become enthused and inspired by the vision of the Sacred Marriage that Heart Yoga opens. With daily practice, however, eventually you will meet resistance. Everyone feels resistance sometimes. Don't judge yourself for it; it's normal. Instead, respond to it skillfully.

When you notice resistance in your yoga practice, simply feel that sensation. Do not identify with it, as if that is all you are. When resistance is in the body and you feel pain, use your breath to explore the edges of the resistance and gently release around it. Sometimes the pain will lessen or dissolve, and then you may move a bit further into it and explore it again. If the sensation is strong, or if it's in a joint rather than in the body of a muscle, you may wish to consider consulting a health professional. Listen deeply to the message of the pain, and respond compassionately.

Mental resistance can be more difficult to unravel. For example, in Dog Pose, you might feel pain in your hamstrings. Your mind may immediately start weaving a story around this sensation, such as, "I'm an athlete, and I'll always have short hamstrings. I don't want to do this. I hate this pose." The ego may be resisting the yoga practice to protect itself against the momentary dissolution that looks like death but is liberation! Embrace resistance with acceptance and practice anyway. Think of the Buddha assaulted by many illusions when he sat all night under the Bodhi Tree and stayed in his seat despite it all. Over time, you learn that you can trust the practice; it's spacious enough to contain everything, even resistance! Learn to be amused at the stratagems the ego devises to try to prevent you from your deepest happiness and realizing your true nature.

Breath

Breath is life itself. It is the basic and most fundamental expression of our life. In Islam, it is God's breath that infuses Adam and births Creation. In Judaism *Ruach,* the breath, signifies the spirit of God that infuses all things. In Christian mystical practice, the Greek Orthodox mystics tell us, the breath and the Holy Spirit are intimately intertwined, since it is the Holy Spirit that creates life and breath. In the teaching of Buddha, the breath, or *prana* in Sanskrit, is called the vehicle of the mind because it is prana that makes our mind move. Buddhist mystics also point out that prana is the subtlest connection between consciousness and matter, the placeless place where they meet in exquisite embrace. Work skillfully with your breath, then, and you will bring peace to your mind and peace to all the cells of your body.

When you begin yoga, don't worry about complicated breathing practices. Simply observe your normal, natural breath. Notice how the breath responds in different postures. You will breathe more quickly when you're in more demanding poses. Your breath will naturally lengthen and grow steadier when the postures begin to be practiced with more ease. As the body relaxes and grows more supple and receptive, the breath will flow more freely. Notice where in the body your breath flows easily and where it feels restricted. Explore the presence of emotions or sensations in these restricted places. Imagine your body as having doors and windows, and picture yourself easing them open with your breath, to let the breath flow more fluidly. Your breath will reveal to you subtle truths about your body and emotions if you keep listening to and observing it.

O friend, understand: the body
is like the ocean,
rich with hidden treasures.

Open your innermost chamber and light its lamp.

Within the body are gardens,
Rare flowers, peacocks, the inner Music;
Within the body a lake of bliss,
On it the white soul-swans take their joy.

—MIRABAI[18]

Ending and Dedicating Your Practice

After you have completed your practice, remember again to be gentle with yourself. The Dalai Lama once told Andrew, "After meditation of any kind you should treat yourself for a while as if you were made of eggshells, or as if you were a parent holding a newborn baby." This is important because this tenderness and kindness with yourself will allow the full effects of the practice to suffuse your whole being and ground you in peace throughout your day. In our experience, in the haste of our busy world, we all need to remember how essential it is after practice to allow a time for our whole being to breathe in its new fullness and peace. Do not let the impatience of the ego and its agendas prevent you from savoring the radiance into which the practice of Heart Yoga has led you. When you do re-enter everyday life, let the wisdom, fluidity, compassion, and spaciousness that your practice brought you pervade your day-to-day experience.

One of the deepest effects you will find from practicing Heart Yoga is that over time, it will heal you in subtle ways of that body-shame and self-dislike that we all carry as products of a materialistic culture. As the realization and experience grows in you of the power of the heart to infuse your whole being and awaken divine love energy in the depths of your cells, you will open to ever increasing self-knowledge and joy. This will reveal to you the deep compassion, fearlessness, and bliss of your authentic nature. The inherent, divinely given qualities of the heart become fully conscious in every aspect of your being. As this awakening deepens, you will find that you will naturally want to serve all sentient beings and see them happy, cherished, and safe. In a time as difficult as ours, letting your natural love overflow as Sacred Activism is the key, not only to your own full self-realization but to the healing that the world so desperately needs on every level.

An essential way of helping yourself out of the ego's inevitable and inveterate narcissism is to remember, both at the beginning *and* at the end of your practice, to dedicate and offer all the joy, insight, and peace you have derived from your practice to the liberation of all beings from suffering and injustice. At first when you do this you may feel self-conscious and not completely convinced that your dedication has any real effect. The mystics of the Sacred Marriage in all traditions tell us two essential things about the reality of the nature of the heart. The first is that all things are interrelated in unimaginably mysterious, exquisite, and transformative ways. The second is that no act of love or thought of being of help to others is ever wasted in a universe interconnected in the bliss of love-consciousness. This means that your slightest authentic intention of wanting to help others travels immediately at a speed faster than the speed of light along all the invisible threads of the web of the Mother-Father. It is received and used immediately by the supreme grace that sustains, underpins, and directs all things. To know this is to know the enormous power that is given to those awakened in the heart, a power to effect deep change through simple acts of giving away all the merits of one's practice, and of all one's actions, to the happiness and liberation of all beings.

We would like to suggest some simple yet inspiring ways of dedicating your practice in this manner. First, before and after your practice, stand in Mountain Pose for some long, calm moments, savoring all the richness and beauty of the presence now vibrant within you. Cupping your hands over your heart, consciously extend to the four directions that richness and that beauty. Spread your arms, imagining that from your open hands streams of golden light travel to all the beings in the different directions, filling them in heart, mind, soul, and body with the radiance of the presence. Imagine this light healing them of whatever suffering is blocking their deepest fulfillment and their realization of the divine within. As you do this, wish all beings liberation from suffering and injustice.

A second visualization you could use at the beginning and end of your practice is to imagine and know in the depths of your being that the sincerity and authenticity of your practice have, through the grace of the Beloved, transformed you into a vast mountain diamond, what the Buddhists call a wish-fulfilling jewel. Many of us are deeply perturbed at the state of the world and have causes we hold especially dear. Choose one cause in the world that breaks your heart—it could be environmental disaster, genocide in Darfur, the plight of animals, or the continuing devastating treatment of women and gay people. Radiating divine light in all directions as a mountain diamond, consciously send that light to all those working tirelessly for the cause you love so that they may have strength, peace, and courage to go on being heroic Sacred Activists, devoted to the future of humanity. You will find that if you do this repeatedly, your own desire to become an active servant of transformation in the world will grow, as will as your compassion and self-realization.

A third practice you can use is to imagine yourself as the Mother or the Father of the universe, and hold the entire world and all its beings to your awakened heart as if it were a small child. Closing your eyes, summon up all your memories of joy and peace during your practice. Bring to focus everything you know about divine and human love. Imagine the world and all its beings that you are holding to your heart to be suffused with the all-healing and all-transforming diamond light of divine consciousness. In a state of faith, confidence, and peace, pray for the peace of the world.

We have found that it is extremely powerful to end this process of dedication with a prayer. We recommend the following three prayers. The first is said daily by the Dalai Lama. He has often spoken of its enormous transformative power.

> I would be a protector for those without protection, a leader for those who journey, and a boat, a bridge, a passage for those desiring the further shore.
>
> For all creatures, I would be a lantern for those desiring a lantern, I would be a bed for those desiring a bed, I would be a slave for those desiring a slave.
>
> I would be for creatures a magic jewel, an inexhaustible jar, a powerful spell, a universal remedy, a wishing tree, and a cow of plenty.
>
> As the earth and other elements are, in various ways, for the enjoyment of innumerable beings dwelling in all of space;
>
> So may I be, in various ways, the means of sustenance for the living beings occupying space, for as long a time as all are not satisfied.
>
> —SHANTIDEVA[19]

Second, Andrew has adapted his favorite prayer of Teresa of Avila for every tradition.

> The Beloved has no body now on Earth but mine.
> The Beloved has no hands on Earth but mine,
> The Beloved has no feet on Earth but mine.
> Mine are the eyes through which the
> Beloved streams compassion to the world.
> Mine are the feet with which the Beloved is to go about healing,
> loving, and serving all beings now.
> Mine are the hands with which the Beloved is to bless all beings.
> May I have the courage to know this Mystery, the faith to give
> myself to it entirely, and the strength to enact its truth in this world,
> And give to its embodiment everything I am and everything I have.
> In the name of the all-compassionate, all-merciful Mother-Father,
> may their will be done, and the world become the garden of the
> golden dancer, the garden of the Sacred Marriage.

A third dedication or prayer to offer at the end of your practice is from Rumi:

> You are glorified in heaven, O subtle Sun!
> Be glorified now on Earth for eternity!
> May the inhabitants of Earth become one in their hearts,
> Unite their plans and designs with the dwellers in heaven!
> All forms of separation and duality will vanish
> For there's only unity in real existence!
> When my spirit recognizes your spirit fully,
> Then the two of us remember being one before
> And we become on Earth like Moses and Aaron,
> Heart-brothers united tenderly like honey and milk.

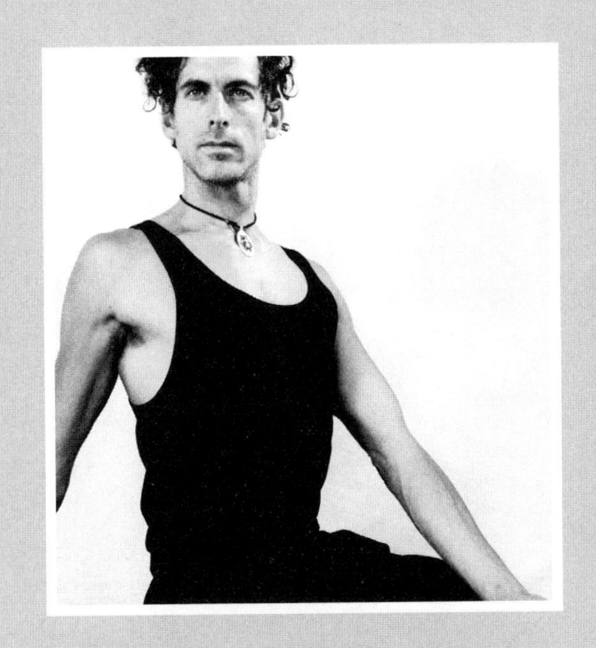

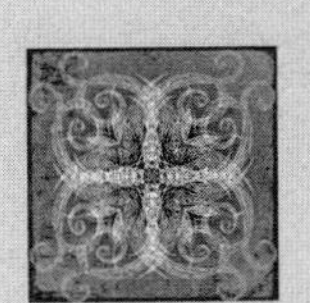 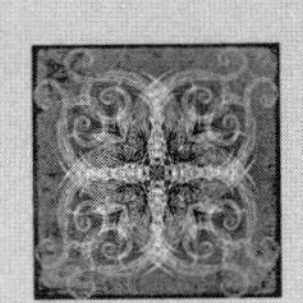 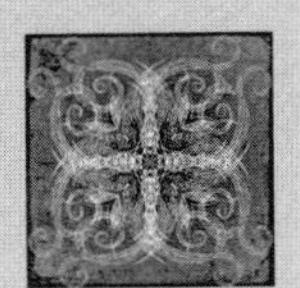

TWO
The Mystical Body

The Dalai Lama explains that "According to Buddhist Vajrayana thought, there is an understanding that our bodies represent microcosmic images of the greater macrocosmic world."[1] In Seyyed Hossein Nasr's brilliant analysis of Islamic mysticism, he states,

> The human also corresponds to the cosmos, not only in the sense of sharing with it the same constituent elements, but in containing in miniature form the whole cosmos. It is by virtue of this correspondence between us as living bodies, soul, and spirit and the cosmos as a whole, which is also alive—having its own "soul" and dominated by the spirit—that we are able to know the cosmos. We also occupy a special and central position in it because of our being the cosmic totality in miniature form, a replica of the Universe, so that in the deepest sense the body of the cosmos is *our* body. Our intimate contact with the forms of nature around us as well as attraction to the beauty of the stars issues not from simple sentimentality but from an inner *sympatheia*, which relates us to all things, a union of essences or "inner breath" to which Rumi refers as *hamdami*, and which joins us, in our mind and body bi-unity, to the world about us and finally to the entire cosmos. This link is, however, much greater than simply the presence of iron in our blood and in rocks. It involves the Spirit, which inbreathes our body, and the cosmos and the Divine Archetype, which our bodies reflect. . . .[2]

Heart Yoga is restoring in full the vision of the body that is central to the ancient wisdom traditions, but which has been obscured for centuries by our addiction to purely scientific explanations of things. When most people who have been brought up in our modern, materialistic society think of consciousness, they imagine it as being somewhere vaguely inside the body. From the mystical point of view, the reality is very different. In this view, the body is "inside" consciousness. In fact, the body is an exquisite crystallization of spiritual and psychic forces. This view is corroborated by the latest discoveries of modern physics, which reveal that matter is light-energy. When the body is consciously experienced as concentrated light-energy, it can be profoundly affected, and a wholly new level of dynamic healing and transformation is accessible.

This is not a truth known only to great yogis; it is actually something that you have already experienced many times. Remember those moments when you have felt great bliss, ecstasy, or sudden rushes of energy through your body. These may have come to you while listening to great music, being outside in the majesty of nature, in the tender joy after lovemaking, or when you felt at one with all Creation. All these are moments when the essential light-energy of the body and your essential nature as crystallized consciousness are revealed to you. These direct experiences allow you to open to the mystery of the subtle anatomy of the body.

The aim of Heart Yoga is not only to make the body healthier and more supple. This yoga also creates an open and spacious foundation to receive the direct transforming energies of the divine light consciousness. Eventually every cell can enter into lucid, joyful, and constantly regenerative communion with its origin.

Grand and majestic though this process is, the principles behind it are very simple. Since the body is in fact concentrated light-energy, it can be worked on directly to astonishing effect by consciousness, using different techniques and forms of awareness of how the light operates. In this way, human beings awaken and attune to the all-pervading reality of divine light-energy, and we can learn to align with this subtle energy and transform our entire being.

Through our studies of the origins of yoga, we have found that yoga philosophy reveals that the transforming experience of embodying light-energy was known at the dawn of yoga. This confirmation has deepened our awe of the yoga tradition. At least four thousand years ago, the Vedic Rishis of India discovered what they called "the great passage," *mahas pathah* (Rig Veda, II.24.6), the world of "the unbroken Light," *Svar.* In the Vedas, we find these words: "Our fathers by their words broke the strong and stubborn places, the Angirasa seers shattered the mountain rock with their cry; they made in us a path to the Great Heaven, they discovered the Day and the sun-world." (1.71.2)

The great evolutionary mystic, Sri Aurobindo, uncovered the key to these words. The "Day and sun-world" that these seers discovered is the divine solar energy released by the marriage of the transcendent and the immanent in the core of every cell. The release of this hidden divine energy acts to realize the potential we already have as "children of the light" to become consciously evolved servants of God in the world. The Vedic sages and Aurobindo understood that by this release of the body's own inherent divine energy, we participate in the evolutionary dance of the divine and attain a new level of consciousness and radical embodied empowerment.

The Vedic Rishis and Aurobindo saw that this solar energy of the Day and sun-world is the fundamental energy of evolution. When we work with it consciously, as Heart Yoga supports, we co-create with the Divine the new level of strength, empowerment, and vision for which the Divine has always destined us. The Divine is at once absolute being and dynamic becoming. The infinite consciousness that we are given as a blessing unites us with the mystery of divine being. The energy of the Day and sun-world, uncovered through Heart Yoga, fuses us consciously with the dynamic evolutionary energy of the divine becoming. When, through the marriage of yoga and mysticism, we join the breadth and peace of the consciousness of infinite being with the experience of the all-transforming vibrant energy of infinite becoming, the full glory of what it means to be divine humans starts to be unveiled in us. The logic of divine transformation begins to birth us into our divine humanity.

The limitation of the ancient patriarchal mystical traditions has been their bias toward transcendence. The Vedic Rishis and Aurobindo, while honoring transcendence, were also aware of its feminine presence in the immanent, as the solar energy within matter. The Sacred Marriage heals the bias of ancient traditions by honoring the full power and majesty of the feminine, and so making available to the human race the complete empowerment of both being and becoming. As Bede Griffiths explains:

> Body and soul are to be transfigured by the divine life and to participate in the divine consciousness. There is a descent of the spirit into matter and a corresponding ascent, by which matter is transformed by the indwelling power of the Spirit and the body is transfigured. In kundalini yoga this is represented as the union of *Shiva* and *Shakti* in the human body. The divine power is represented as coiled up like a serpent at the base of the spine. This divine energy has to be led through the seven *chakras,* or centers of psychic energy, until it reaches the thousand-petaled lotus at the crown of the head. Then Shiva, who is pure consciousness, unites with Shakti, the divine energy in nature, and body and soul are transformed. This is very different from the yoga of Patanjali, where consciousness *(purusha)* is separated from nature *(prakriti)* and enjoys the bliss of isolation *(kaivalya).* Yet both these yogas have their place. There must be a movement of ascent to pure consciousness, a detachment from all the moods of nature, a realization of the Self in its eternal Ground beyond space and time. But then there must also be a movement of descent, by which the Spirit enters into the depths of matter and raises it to a new mode of existence, in which it becomes the medium of a spiritual consciousness.[3]

In this book you will discover the Heart Yoga practices that we find most effective in aligning the inherent light-energy of the body with the all-pervading divine light consciousness. By uniting the ancient practical instructions of yoga with mystical techniques and exercises that work directly with divine energy consciousness, a potent crucible is created for the divinization of the entire being. This fusion of the sacred technology of yoga with that of mystical transformation invokes and engenders a new evolutionary energy, which births a fully integrated and divinely empowered human being.

The language and imagery of mystical traditions and esoteric anatomy are often used in this book to convey the beauty and wonder of the asana practice. This will help you experience deeper levels of the subtlety of the mystery of the light-body. When yoga is experienced in this consciously divine and mystical way, even the simplest gestures become prayers, every breath is an act of love, and every asana helps us birth the divine in the human.

Here is one simple exercise you can use to celebrate the Sacred Marriage we are experiencing in Heart Yoga, and so, in the reality of your mystical body. Imagine sending roots down into the earth through your feet and legs. Find the axis in the center of your body joining your tailbone and the crown of your head. Align your spine, balancing the bones of your spine one by one lightly upon each other, so that your muscles do not have to overwork to support you.

When your body is precisely aligned, the core channel may feel empty, as if all of you had dispersed into shining space. As the Vastusutra Upanishad said, "Getting the limbs along proper lines is praised like the knowledge of Brahman."[4]

Into this opening channel, breathe down into the depths of the earth, and when you exhale, let the exhalation dissolve slowly up and out through the crown of your head into infinite space. You may begin to experience your body as the mysteriously vibrating channel between earth and sky. This will awaken you to the experience of your body fusing the density of the earth with the luminosity of the light in a dynamic dance.

Now imagine matter and light dancing together in interlocking golden spirals all through your body. Gaze at every part of your body with compassion and wonder, the way you would look at a newborn baby.

Continue to visualize yourself as a light-body, surrounded by luminous fields of light. This will build a sense of wonder and infinite respect, both for you and for all other embodied beings. Experience your body as porous light matter, open to and dancing subtly with the entire cosmos.

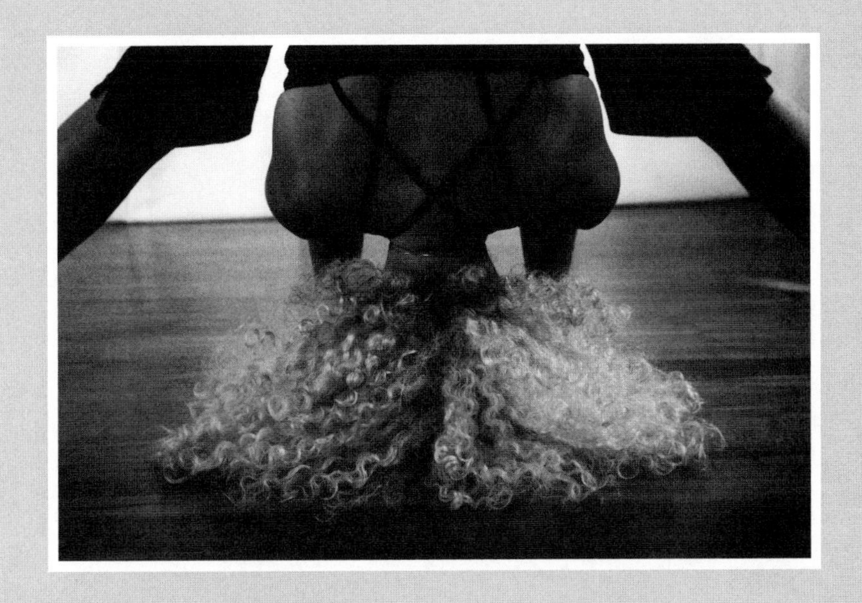

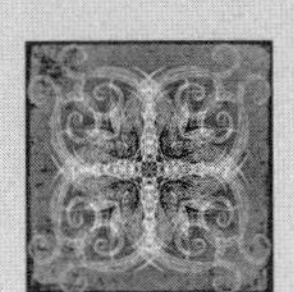 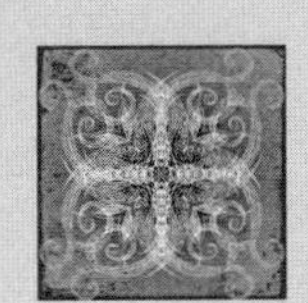 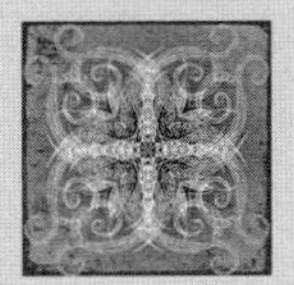

THREE

Heart Yoga: The Sacred Marriage of Yoga and Mysticism

The body
is like an ocean,
rich with hidden treasures.

Open its innermost chamber and light its lamp.

—MIRABAI[1]

Many teachers and students in the yoga community are now searching for and discovering luminous new ways of deepening the body's experience of spirit. They intuit that it is this experience of dynamic unity that will inspire, encourage, and strengthen people to meet the challenges of our time. Many mystical teachers and students also are aware that this moment in history demands not only spiritual knowledge but a divinely embodied strength and a capacity for compassionate action. They are turning toward yoga as a way of discovering the new grounding inspiration that they need.

Heart Yoga is our attempt to fuse both these longings and aspirations. Our quietly revolutionary work is born from a deep belief that the healing revelation for our time is that of the Sacred Marriage. In most of the world's mystical traditions the universe is conceived as a dynamic dance of opposites, the most profound of which are masculine and feminine: spirit and matter. Their electric unity leads to a new level of both mystical knowledge and embodied physical energy. We believe this is essential for the most empowered evolution of the human race. The Sacred Marriage is the living unity of heaven and earth, heart and mind, body and soul. The inner experience of this marriage engenders a transformed human being, one who is simultaneously open to the transcendent and able to create and work for radical change in the immanent.

The most crucial aspect of the Sacred Marriage for our time is what we call Sacred Activism. We believe that only intense and deep mystical love, strength, and passion, combined with a commitment to sustained transformative action, can now preserve the planet. This fusion of body and soul enables people to find the luminous energy, calm, and power that they will need in order to become Sacred Activists and give birth to a new world.

We believe that the unity of spirit, body, heart, and mind that all human beings are longing for can be powerfully achieved through the union of simple yoga asanas with simple spiritual practices from many traditions, which we present in this book. This union creates an ecstatic and passionate experience of the Divine, inspiring people to directly taste the glory of their true spiritual nature and to embody its power in the authenticity of their humanity.

The Sacred Marriage of the essence of yoga traditions with mystical traditions is especially designed for our challenging times. We feel that the most profound way of staying awake, passionate, and grounded comes from the unity of body and soul. It provides the continuous peaceful strength and stable power needed to sustain loving action in the world.

The fusion of yoga and mysticism fulfills the longing of many yoga teachers and students for a deeper spiritual meaning to their practice, while also satisfying the desire of many mystics for a greater and deeper experience of embodiment. Heart Yoga brings together the world of yoga and the world of mystical seeking and practice.

We pray that all those who open to this innovative and exciting blend of ancient teachings will become radiant with a renewed commitment to spiritual growth and service to all beings, empowered with the practices they need to sustain their lives in the marriage of love, peace, and sacred passion.

> The spirit has made itself matter in order to place itself there as an instrument for the well-being ... and joy, of created beings, for a self-offering of universal physical utility and service.
>
> —SRI AUROBINDO[2]

Yoga Practice Sequence to Celebrate the Sacred Marriage

- Cross-legged Sitting – *Sukhasana*
- Downward-facing Dog Pose – *Adho Mukha Svanasana*

- Mountain Pose – *Tadasana*
- Sun Salutations – *Surya Namaskar*
- Tree Pose – *Vrksasana*
- Triangle Pose – *Trikonasana*
- Wide-legged Standing Forward Bend – *Prasarita Padottanasana*
- Squatting Pose – *Malasana*
- Bridge Pose – *Setu Bandhasana*
- Knees to Chest to Reclined Back Twist – *Jathara Parivartanasana*
- Cross-legged Sitting – *Sukhasana*
- Cross-legged Sitting Twist – *Pavritta Sukhasana*
- Child's Pose – *Adho Mukha Virasana*
- Corpse Pose – *Savasana*

This sequence of yoga poses embodies and celebrates the experience of the union of transcendence and immanence, heaven and earth, soul and body, masculine and feminine. All the seeming opposites dance as One in the human/divine temple of the body/mind/heart.

Cross-Legged Sitting
Sukhasana

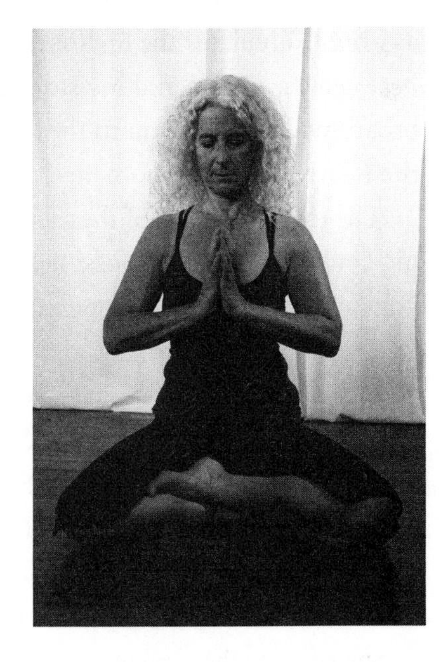

Sit in a position that is comfortable for you, elevating your hips on a cushion. Begin your practice in a sacred manner by lighting a candle, for example. Offer the fruits of your practice for the benefit of all beings, or dedicate your practice to something that is important to you. In whatever way spontaneously arises for you, ask to be gathered body, mind, heart, and soul into the dynamic ecstasy of the union of transcendence and immanence.

The continual changes of the flex of the mouth, and around the eyes,
The skin, the sunburnt shade, freckles, hair,
The curious sympathy one feels when feeling with the hand the naked meat of the body,
The circling rivers of the breath, and breathing it in and out,
The beauty of the waist, and thence of the hips, and thence downward toward the knees,
The thin red jellies within you or within me, the bones and the marrow in the bones,
The exquisite realization of health;
O I say these are not the parts and poems of the body only, but of the soul,
O I say now these are the soul.

—WALT WHITMAN[1]

Bring your awareness to your breath. Allow it to guide the movement of your practice. Feel it flowing deep within you, like an underground river. Following your breath is itself a form of prayer. Breath, known in Sanskrit as *prana,* circulates the life force and is the most obvious and natural bridge between the visible and invisible. Honoring and deeply connecting with the breath will awaken you to the natural interdependence of the absolute and the relative in every moment.

The mystical secret of the sacred marriage of body with Self, which breathing consciously makes possible, has been exquisitely expressed by the great yoga master, B. K. S. Iyengar:

> Inhalation is the extension and expansion of the Self *(Purusa)*. With the help of the in-breath, the Self embraces its sheaths up to the skin of the body, like a lover embracing his beloved. Retention after inhalation is the union of the lover with his beloved. In exhalation, the Self, via the out-breath, takes the beloved to his home where, in her turn, the beloved embraces her lover, the Self. Retention after exhalation is the beloved uniting with the lover in total surrender to the supreme.[2]

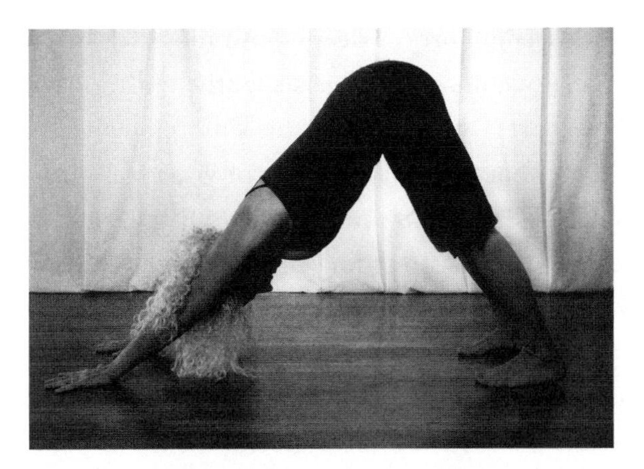

Downward-facing Dog Pose
Adho Mukha Svanasana

Coming to the hands and knees, gently rock the pelvis back and forth a few times, releasing the spine. On an exhalation, lift your tailbone to the sky, while firmly rooting down to earth through the four limbs. Earth and sky unite in the body as lover and beloved. Stay here for a few breaths, and then walk your feet forward and rise up to standing. See page 69 for detailed instruction.

Mountain Pose
Tadasana

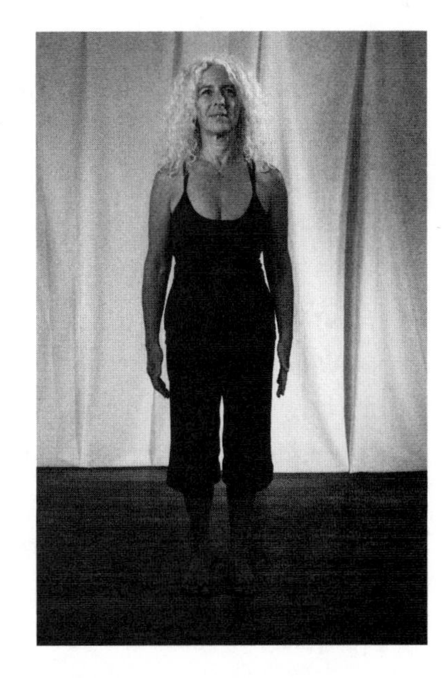

Inspired by the vision of the holiness of breathing, stand in the majesty and simplicity of the Mountain Pose, *Tadasana.* Embed your feet deeply into the earth, rooting yourself in this precious present moment. Slowly open the palms of your hands, symbolically letting go of whatever you've been holding onto in your life. Let tension, grasping, and stress fall away like golden wax rolling down a burning candle.

Feel your feet extending roots deeply into the earth beneath you. Stand with your big toes touching, your heels slightly apart, or with feet parallel and a few inches apart (whichever way feels more balanced to you).

Sense the deep connection of the soles of your feet with the floor, as if they were kissing the earth. Lift and spread your toes, and when you place them down, feel the energy streaming through each toe from its base to its tip. Observe your feet connecting you directly to earth, and feel their aliveness. Imagine you're making a footprint in wet clay. Notice how after some time of sinking into the earth, you will feel a soft, rebounding sensation of energy rising from the earth up through the arches of your feet, as if you were standing on a quivering trampoline. This energy pulses up through the core of your strong and steady legs, and is transformed into a fluid dance inside your pelvis.

Allow your pelvis to rock slightly, until it finds its innate balance and feels spacious and empty. Notice the sensation of energy breathing up the front of your spine from the warm cave of your belly. Feel the lightness of your breath expanding from the airiness of your chest and the vastness of the space around your heart.

> Awake, my dear
> Be kind to your sleeping heart
> Take it out into the vast fields of Light
> And let it breathe . . .
>
> —HAFIZ[3]

Sun Salutations

Surya Namaskar

Notice how these fields of light pour into your chest and head, streaming out into your hands and permeating and illuminating every cell of your body.

Bowing your head slightly and softening your eyes, mindfully draw your hands together in front of your heart, into a position of prayer. This is the *Namaste* position, and it signifies the divine within you honoring the divine

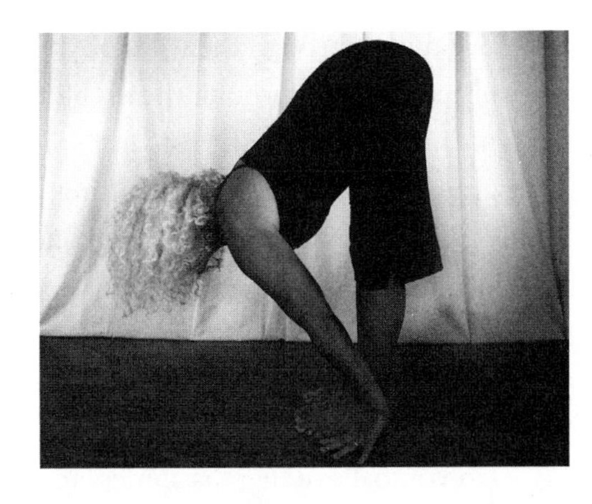

all around you. From this place of devotion, each movement flows like a prayer throughout your body. Inhale, and lift your arms above you, radiating joy and gratitude for this experience of the sacred union of matter and spirit.

Exhale, and sweep your hands down to the floor or to your legs, bending your knees to protect your back. Ground the joyous energy dancing through you as an offering to Mother Earth. Step one foot back, and keeping your heart lifted to radiate your devotion, come into a lunge position. Step the other foot back, balancing evenly on the hands and feet, the spine elongated in plank position. Then release the knees to the ground and lengthen your body onto the earth, melting down into the earth like a young child softening into her mother's body. Alternatively, you can hover above the earth in a strong push-up position.

With your hands under your shoulders, press the hands down and gently curl your spine up slightly, lifting your heart. Notice how it is suffused with the warm nourishment that resting on earth has given you. Lift up to your hands and knees, and slide your sitting bones back to your heels, releasing into Child's Pose (see page 51); or let your sitting bones rise up and come to Downward-facing Dog Pose, where the body is in the shape of an inverted V. Hands and feet are firmly rooted on earth, the tailbone lifts toward the sky, while the crown of the head releases toward the earth (see page 69 for more detailed instructions). Bend your knees here if it feels appropriate, taking a few breaths, hands and feet evenly balanced on earth, spine elongating. Feel your identity and kinship with all four-legged animals.

Exhale, and step forward into the lunge again, and then bring your other foot forward so that you return to a standing forward bend. Allow your head to release completely and let your thoughts pour out like water onto the earth.

Move down through the soles of your feet, lifting up through the arches of your feet and up through the arch of your pelvic floor. Slowly roll up to standing, aligning the bones of your spine lightly on top of each other. Float your arms up above your head, lifting your heart in devotion. Return your hands to prayer position in front of your heart for a few breaths. Then allow your arms to return to your sides, coming again into the majesty of *Tadasana.* Root your entire being in the unshakeable power, steadiness, balance, and peace of the mountain.

> Do you believe there is someplace
> That will make the soul less thirsty?
> In that great absence you will find nothing.
> Be strong then, and enter into your own body.
> There you have a solid place for your feet.
> Think about it carefully!
> Don't go off somewhere else.
> Kabir says this: Just throw away all thoughts of imaginary things,
> And stand firm in that which you are.
>
> —KABIR[4]

Tree Pose

Vrksasana

From the stability of *Tadasana,* imagine that you are a grand and ancient redwood tree, with roots that descend and explore deep into the Mother. Experience this vast network of roots that anchors you, and allow that grounding power to percolate up through your feet and legs.

Now shift your weight to your right foot and allow your left foot to rise, placing the sole of your left foot as high up as possible on the inside of your right leg. If it is difficult to maintain your balance, stand by a wall. Notice how balance is never a fixed point but is always a subtle and spontaneous response to each moment.

From the strong, grounded earthiness of your feet and legs, turn your

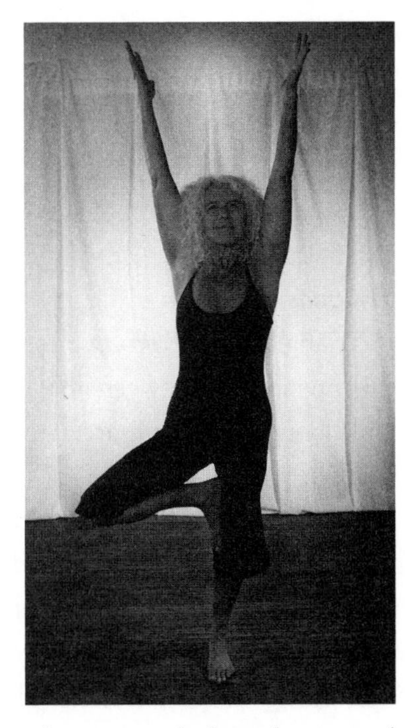

palms out and lift your hands to your heart in prayer position (Namaste). Imagine the rooted Mother Earth energy like red light coursing up your legs, through the watery dance of your belly into your heart. Imagine spacious Father Sky energy like a golden light streaming down through the crown of your head into your heart. Visualize these lights melting ecstatically into each other in the sacred temple of your heart center, dancing in millions of red-gold fire circles that ignite all the cells of your body.

What you are directly experiencing now is the truth of the embodiment of the light. You feel the union of the feminine Shakti power that fills you from below, with the masculine Shiva power that enters you from the crown chakra above, and the ecstatic empowerment of their marriage in the shrine of your heart. Slowly release your hands back to prayer position.

Return to *Tadasana,* experiencing the union that you embody in every cell. Repeat *Vrksasana* (Tree Pose) on the other side, receiving the love of Mother Earth, while opening to the light of Father Sky.

Express the blessing and joy of the Sacred Marriage as you release your arms above you, letting bliss radiate its soft fiery healing power in all directions, while you remain deeply rooted in the support of the earth below. Your body is now a Divine Conduit, the dancing ground of the God and Goddess!

I honor the union of Shiva and Shakti,
who devour this world of name and form
like a sweet dish.
All that remains is the One.
Embracing each other

They merge into One,
As darkness merges with the light
At the breaking of dawn.
—JNANESHWAR[5]

Triangle Pose
Trikonasana

In Triangle Pose *(Trikonasana)* we celebrate and express the mystery of being the intersection between absolute and relative, heaven and earth, the divine child born from the marriage of the transcendent father and the embodied mother.

Step your feet a wide distance apart (one meter or more), embedding them deeply into the ground. Spread your arms wide, at shoulder height, palms down. Elongate from the front of your heart all the way into your middle fingers, and from the back of your heart, between your shoulder blades, out into your little fingers. In the Chinese medicine system, this movement opens the heart and pericardium meridians, thereby releasing the healing flow of energy from the heart and irradiating the whole body-mind with it.

Rest your arms on this flowing line of energy as if they were floating on clouds, rather than gripping onto them from your shoulders. Listen to the dancing dialog between your tailbone and the crown of your head, as spaces open between the bones of your spine. Be aware of your rootedness on earth as well as your soaring connection with the sky. Feel how vital energy radiates evenly from your core in all the five directions of the legs, arms, and head like a starfish.

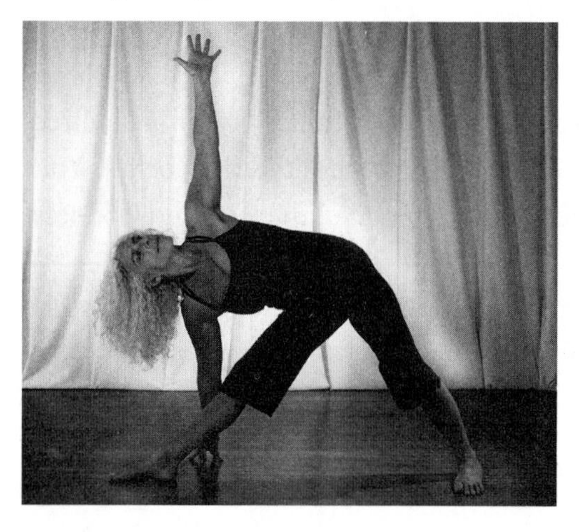

Turn your left foot in slightly and your right foot out 90 degrees, keeping your body facing forward. Inhale, lifting the sides of your waists; exhale and lengthen over to the right side, placing your right hand on a block or your leg for support, while lifting up through the left arm into your fingertips. Balance evenly through your arms and legs, as you elongate from your tailbone to the crown of your head.

The sacred architecture of the Triangle position embodies in a simple and directly accessible way the triune mystery or mystery of the three: the father, mother, and child, the transcendent, immanent, and creation. In the Christian formulation, the triangle symbolizes the Father, Son, and Holy Spirit, in which the Holy Spirit is the mother force of love. In this pose the body itself symbolizes this mystery by creating a variety of triangles.

Inhale, letting your breath lead you up through your top arm, and repeat Triangle Pose to the other side. Feel a sensation of ease and steadiness flowing throughout your body. Stay on this side the same amount of time, experiencing your body as an open channel between Earth and Heaven, firmly rooted on Earth, and opening like a flower of light into heaven.

Wide-legged Standing Forward Bend
Prasarita Padottanasana

In Standing Forward Bend we marry the strength of the immanent, the body, with surrender to the transcendent spirit, allowing the whole body-mind to be filled with the sacred power of this union.

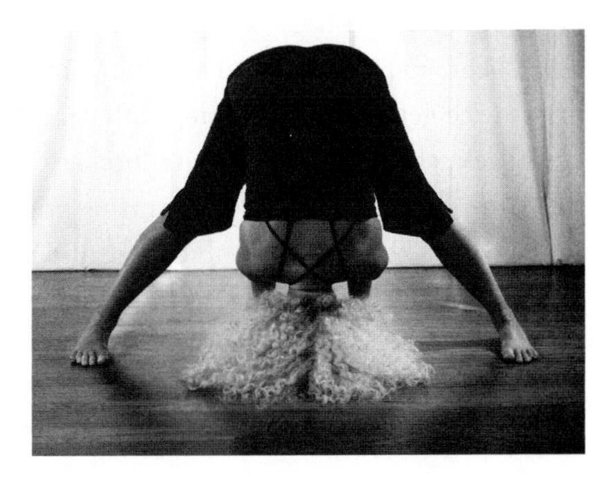

Step your feet a wide distance apart and turn them parallel. Take your hands to the tops of your thighs and slowly move your thighs back, feeling the earthiness of your legs. Let your pelvis release forward over the tops of your thighbones, elongating your spine and shining your heart energy forward. You can put your fingertips onto a block, or place your hands on the floor beneath your shoulders. If you feel any strain in your back or knees, bend your knees or come up.

Allow your spine to release into a crescent moon shape, blending the lunar, receptive energy of your spine with the solar, dynamic energy of your legs.

Enjoy the steadiness of your legs supporting the surrender of your spine: the marriage within your body of strength and softness. Your lower body is firmly grounded while your upper body flows over like a waterfall.

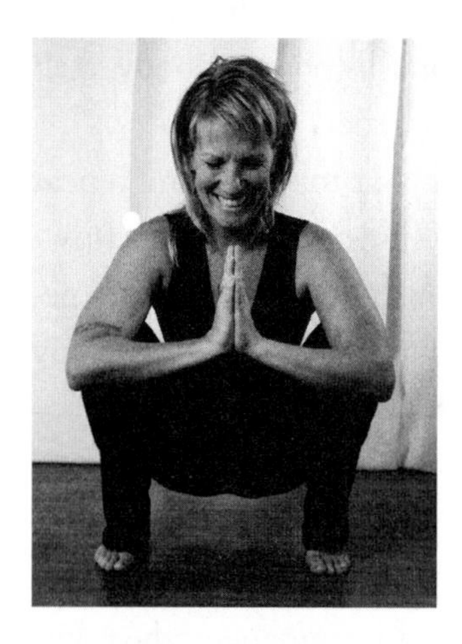

Squatting Pose
Malasana

Now mindfully walk your feet together until they are about hip width apart. Release your sitting bones down toward the floor and come to a squatting position. You may place a folded blanket or low foam block under your heels for balance. Notice the openness of your pelvic floor as the first chakra receives the energy of Mother Earth.

Bridge Pose
Setu Bandhasana

From squatting, roll the sit bones down to the floor. Lie down with your knees bent, your feet parallel and hip width apart. For a few breaths, experiment with gentle pelvic rocking. Inhale, and fill your chest, gently arching your back while releasing your tailbone to the floor. Exhale, and allow your low back to melt into the floor, curling your tailbone slightly. Listen to the subtle dialog between the pubic bone and the tailbone.

On an exhalation, let the lifting of your tailbone draw your hips off the floor, keeping your belly soft and quiet. Your feet and legs stay steady, your hips moving toward your legs, while your chest rises up. Move your arms

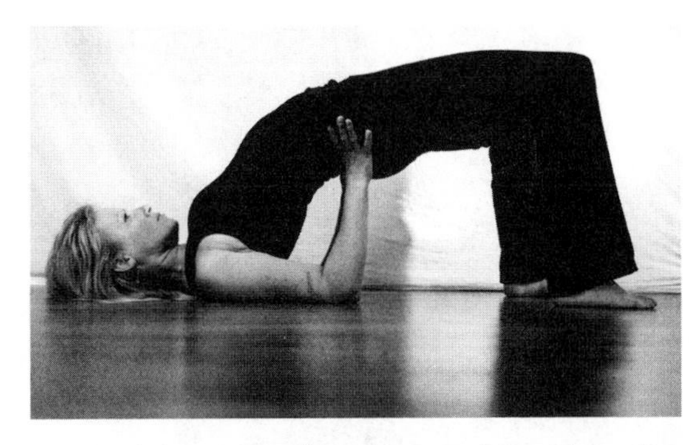

under your back and down toward the earth, rolling your shoulders underneath you.

While lifting your chest, lengthen your hands toward your heels, or interlock your fingers, or place your hands under your back (avoid this latter hand position if you have a wrist injury). Rather than pushing the spine up into the body, move down through your feet, legs, hands, and arms, feeling their bright strength. Allow your spine to relax into a gently rounded crescent moon. In this pose you experience the body celebrating its inherent nature as a bridge between earth and sky, as a child of the Mother-Father. Beginning with the space between your shoulder blades and ending with the tailbone, gradually roll your back down to earth. Repeat a few times.

Try this position with a bolster under your hips and lower shoulder blades, while the tops of your shoulders lightly touch the floor, your arms out to the sides, palms up. Your knees are bent and your feet stand on the floor. Close your eyes and relax here, feeling your body resting on earth, while your heart opens wide to the transcendent sky. Follow your breath, the bridge that marries Body and Self.

> Thinkers, listen, tell me what you know of that is not inside
> the soul?
> Take a pitcher full of water and set it down on the water—
> Now it has water inside and water outside.
> We mustn't give it a name,
> Lest silly people start talking again about the body and the soul.
> If you want the truth, I'll tell you the truth
> Listen to the secret sound, the real sound, which is inside you
>
> —KABIR[6]

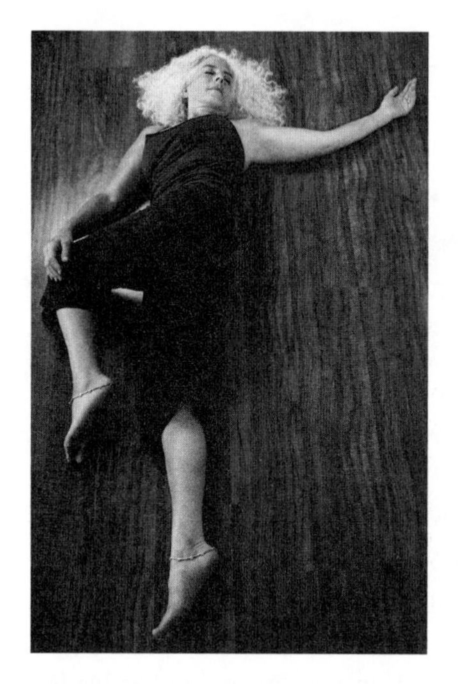

Knees to Chest to Reclined Back Twist
Jathara Parivartanasana
Remaining on your back, exhale and hug your right knee to your chest. Roll your knee across your body and rest it on a pillow, placing your left hand lightly on top of it. Take your right hand to your low back and lengthen your spine. Release your right arm behind you and enjoy this luxurious opening, inhaling into your heart, and exhaling your heart energy out through your right hand as an offering to the world. Slowly return to center, again hugging the right knee to your chest. Repeat on the other side.

Salt gives up its salty taste
To become one with the ocean;
I gave up my individual self
And became
Shiva and Shakti.

When the covering is removed,
The air inside a plantain tree
Merges with the air outside.
And this is how I honor Shiva and Shakti—
By removing all separation and
becoming one with them.
—JNANESHWAR[7]

Come back to the center, hugging your knees to your chest, and then slowly come up to a sitting position.

Cross-Legged Sitting
Sukhasana

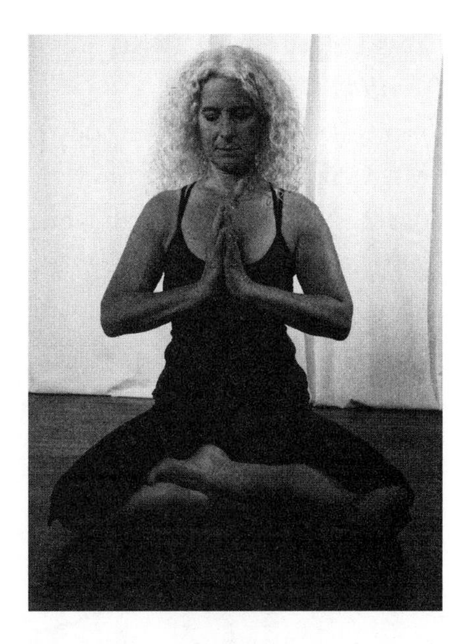

Elevate your sitting bones on a folded blanket or meditation cushion, so that your hips are higher than your knees. Sit groundedly and majestically on the earth, feeling your feet and legs rooting into the earth, while opening your crown chakra to the sky. Imagine the core channel of your body opening like a hollow bamboo to let the divine light flow through. Be open like a bamboo flute, and listen to the song of your own body.

Balance evenly between your two sitting bones, tailbone and pubic bone, mapping those four bones like geographical landmarks within the world of your body. Notice how as your energy descends toward the earth, a corresponding energy rebounds and rises up through the core channel of your body.

With each exhalation, as your diaphragm floats up, your pelvic floor also domes up into your body like a parachute rising. As you exhale, your belly scoops up toward the back of your diaphragm, which also rises. Your heart energy expands while your mind quiets. Notice the alignment between the floor of your pelvis and the crown of your head, and the subtle dialog between them.

It is natural that the cross-legged sitting position is often chosen as a position for meditation, for the meditation on the Infinite that Patanjali said was essential to yoga (Yoga Sutras, II-47) can flow with ease in this position. It both incarnates and enshrines, in perfect balance, the marriage of the groundedness of the embodied with the openness to the transcendent.

Cross-Legged Sitting Twist
Pavritta Sukhasana
Locate the axis inside your body between the pelvic floor and the top of your head. Gently, beginning from your belly, begin to turn toward the right. Root your legs down to the earth while allowing your spine to rise up to the sky. Consciously follow the energy ascending your spine, as if you were ascending, step by step, a spiral staircase to the heavens.

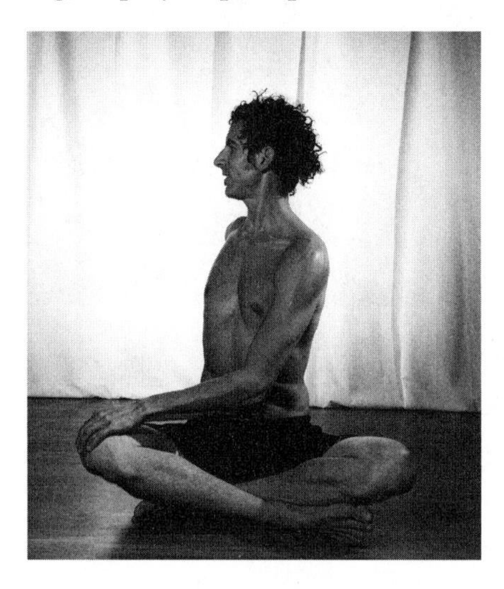

Bring your right hand behind you, sending its roots down into the earth, while your left hand rests on your right thigh. Elongate your spine with each inhalation, and release gradually into the twist with each exhalation. Stay for a few breaths, and then slowly return to center. Rest for a few breaths before exploring the other side. Rather than pushing into the twist, just soften and relax. Experience your skin unraveling and your mind dissolving.

> Walk to the well.
> Turn as the earth and the moon turn,
> Circling what they love.
> Whatever circles comes from the center.
> —RUMI[8]

Slowly return to cross-legged sitting and notice the subtly charged energy infusing your body from the cross-legged twist.

Child's Pose
Adho Mukha Virasana
Come to a kneeling position, slightly widening your knees. Sink your feet,

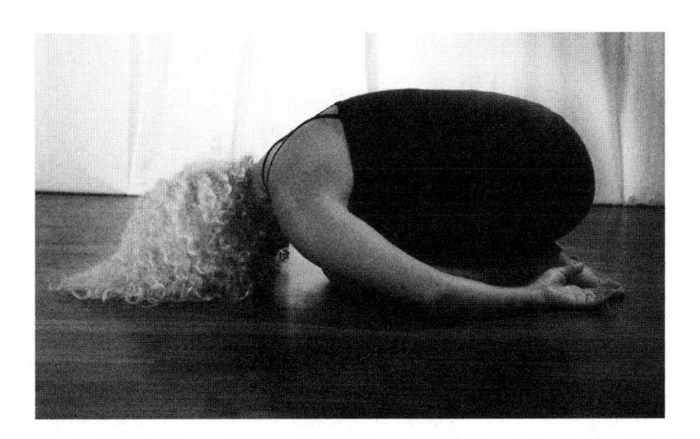

shins, and thighs down into the earth while gently lifting your belly and heart. With an exhalation, slowly release your ribs onto your thighs, resting your hands by your feet, palms soft like a baby's hands. Rest your forehead on your mat or on a bolster, curled into the position of the embryo.

Relax in this position of prayer, melting into the strong loving arms of Mother Earth beneath you. Notice how your breath naturally flows into the backs of your lungs, which open your back ribs like feathers, and widen and release your kidneys. Let your back body open like spreading wings, lifting you into the spaciousness of Father Sky around and above you. With each breath, open every cell to the marriage of the Mother's warm energy rising from the earth with the blessing of the Father's infinite protection from above.

In the Child's Pose for the Sacred Marriage practice, you surrender your inner body into the nurturing tenderness of Mother Earth, while opening your back body to receive the protective blessing of Father Sky raining down upon you as light-energy from above. You can experience in your body, as the great Indian mystic Kabir was said to affirm, "The formless absolute is my Father, and God with form is my Mother."[9] In Child's Pose you incarnate, enshrine, and birth the Sacred Marriage of formlessness and form.

Let go now of any need to do anything or be anybody, letting your entire being fill with gratitude and praise for Mother Earth and Father Sky. Let every cell of your body absorb this timeless prayer from the most ancient of Yogic texts, the Rig Veda:

High Truth, unyielding Order, Consecration,
Ardor and Prayer and Holy Ritual
Uphold the Earth; may she, the ruling Mistress
Of what has been and what will come to be,
for us spread wide a limitless domain.

Impart to us those vitalizing forces
That come, O Earth, from deep within your body,
Your central point, your navel; purify us wholly.
The Earth is mother; I am son (daughter) of Earth.
The Rain-giver is my father; may he shower on us
blessings! . . .

Instill in me abundantly that fragrance,
O Mother Earth, which emanates from you
And from your plants and waters, that sweet perfume
That all celestial beings are wont to emit,
And let no enemy ever wish us ill! . . .

Peaceful and fragrant, gracious to the touch,
May Earth, swollen with milk, her breasts overflowing,
Grant me her blessing together with her milk! . . .
—RIG VEDA 5.84[10]

Corpse Pose
Savasana
Given the magnificence of what *Savasana* can offer you, it is important that the body rests in perfect alignment so that you can surrender into the peace of this pose.

Begin on your back with your knees bent and your feet flat on the ground. Place your elbows on the floor next to your ribs, with your palms up, and

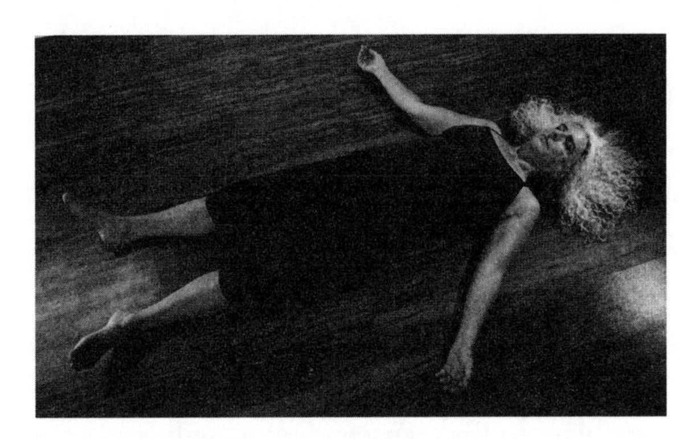

roll your shoulder blades down toward your waist while widening them sideways. Lift your pelvis, curling your tailbone toward your pubic bone and elongating your lumbar spine. As you lower your pelvis onto the ground, draw the flesh of your buttocks toward your heels.

Elongate your legs out from the hip joints onto the ground, letting your feet fall sideways. Allow your legs to drop from the pelvis and toward the floor, feeling them sink into the earth like a fallen tree decomposing into the forest floor. Release your arms along the ground, your palms gently turned upwards. Align your legs and arms, so they are equidistant from the midline of the body. Lengthen your neck so that your chin is slightly lower than your forehead. You will find that this quiets the frontal lobes of your brain.

Care for yourself lovingly as you settle into *Savasana.* You may want to place a small support under your cervical spine, to help relax your neck. A blanket rolled under your knees can release low back tension. Let your pelvic organs float within the cauldron of your pelvic basin. Be sure that you are warm enough to relax completely. Using a light eye pillow over your eyes helps you to relax and soften them, and the mind to settle into silence. A folded blanket on top of your legs helps them melt back into the earth. As the eyes and legs begin to let go, watch whatever thoughts arise, and without attachment, release them also. Feel your muscles melting away from the bones, and the bones sinking deeply into the vast loving arms of Mother Earth.

No one has described *Savasana* more sumptuously and reverently than B. K. S. Iyengar. He states, "*Savasana* is about shedding.... We have many skins, sheaths, thoughts, prejudices, preconceptions, ideas, memories and projects for the future. *Savasana* is a shedding of all these skins, to see how glossy and gorgeous, serene and aware is the beautiful rainbow-colored snake who lies within."[11]

In *Savasana,* we relax completely, our arms and legs outstretched on the ground. We are sustained and upheld by the immanent, while in expansive peace we open ourselves to the transcendent, slowly and gently entering the timeless marriage.

Savasana, as Iyengar describes,

> ... is about relaxation ... to relax is to cut tension. To cut tension is to cut the threads that bind us to identity. To lose identity is to find out who we are not ... As you are lying on the earth in *Savasana,* do you not, when the posture is harmonious and balanced, feel both present and formless? When you feel present yet formless, do you not feel an absence of specific identity? You are there, but who is there? ... *Savasana* is being without was, being without will be. It is being without anyone who is. Is it any wonder that it is the most difficult asana and the door to non-dualist meditation and the cosmic fusion of Samadhi?[12]

Samadhi could be described as the ultimate experience of the Sacred Marriage, for in Samadhi all name, form, and sensation vanish into the calm bliss of the union of the Mother-Father within us and the revelation of our true self.

> I am the infinite ocean.
>
> When thoughts spring up,
> The wind freshens, and like waves
> A thousand worlds arise.

But when the wind falls,
The trader sinks with his ship.

On the boundless ocean of my being
He founders,
And all the worlds with him.

But O how wonderful!

I am the unbounded deep
In whom all living things
Naturally arise,
Rush against each other playfully,
And then subside.

—FROM *THE ASHTAVAKRA GITA*[13]

As the body grows still, bring awareness to the senses. Your eyes grow ever softer, dropping away from the inside of your eyelids, nestling deeper into the eye sockets. The inner gaze streams toward the heart center. Your inner ears relax and listen to the sound of your heartbeat. All the senses awaken to an acute and crystalline sensitivity.

Mind set free in the Dharma-realm,
I sit at the moon-filled window
Watching the mountains with my ears,
Hearing the stream with open eyes.
Each molecule preaches perfect law,
Each moment chants true sutra:
The most fleeting thought is timeless.
A single hair's enough to stir the sea.

—SHUTAKU[14]

Your forehead broadens as the eyebrows drop, and the space between them opens and relaxes. The skin around the temples softens back toward your ears, the cheekbones relax, and your lower jaw drops slightly, the lips barely touching. The root of the tongue releases and the mouth cavity widens.

Notice the skin becoming more porous, transparent, and translucent. The light inside freely radiates out in all directions, and the light outside permeates you from all directions. As the shell of your body falls away, there is a delicate interpenetration of self and world. The skin releases, the weight of the body melts into the earth, and the mind expands to the cosmos. All boundaries separating inner and outer softly dissolve and evaporate.

As the boundaries of the body continue dissolving and evaporating, the edges of the personality begin to crumble. Begin to let go now, of any beliefs, opinions, judgments, or fears that separate you from the vast self that is now being unveiled.

Feel yourself sinking back ever deeper into the embrace of the Mother, like a child nestling back into her mother's arms. Surrender to the warmth of the earth beneath you. Feel the pull of gravity drawing you down into Her core, and the power of Her great love uniting you to Her and to all creation. . . .

When the body has completely relaxed, gently draw your attention to the breath. Observe how the inhalations and exhalations naturally begin to lengthen in *Savasana*. Notice the growing pause at the end of the inhalation; absorb and savor its fullness. Follow the exhalation to its completion, watching it float away into emptiness. Observe the growing pause at the end of the exhalation, and rest in its peace. In awe and wonder, let each breath take you deeper into the mystery of trust. Gratefully deepen into the earth with each inhalation, while expanding into the spaciousness with each exhalation. The body is now vibrant, uniting in lucid, luminous balance earth and sky, feminine and masculine, dark and light, immanent and transcendent, embodying the essence of yoga in this union, this Sacred Marriage.

The cup of the body opens completely to receive the wine of divine love pouring into it from all directions.

The wine of divine grace is limitless
All limits come only from the faults of the cup.
Moonlight floods the whole sky from horizon to horizon.
How much it can fill your room depends on its windows.
Grant a great dignity, my friend, to the cup of your life.
Love has designed it to hold its eternal wine.
—RUMI[15]

Returning from *Savasana*

Rest in *Savasana* as long as you wish. When you are ready to return from *Savasana,* gently return your awareness to your breath. From the stillness, silence, and spaciousness of *Savasana,* sense the breath moving slowly toward you, like a breeze drifting across a vast meadow. Notice how the breath flows toward your body from the infinite, moving from the universal consciousness to the individual consciousness.

With the body now so deeply relaxed and receptive, you can feel your breath flowing smoothly and easily. Bathe yourself in this healing breath, letting it permeate every cell of your body. Observe your breath washing over your body and then flowing away. Each breath arises from and dissolves back into the source. The breath is a golden thread weaving you into the web of all life. Breathing in this peace, equanimity, ease, and relaxation, spread it evenly throughout your body, and beyond your body into the world. Extend this peace out and offer it to the people around you and to the world beyond.

From this expansive awareness, slowly begin to notice the sounds around you, feeling the air on your face, and the shape of your body resting on the earth beneath you. When you feel ready, and fully present in this precious moment, slowly roll to your right side, feeling the whole earth supporting you as you turn. Be aware of your movement from *Savasana,* Corpse Pose (the position of death), to the position of birth. Each moment is a new birth, a fresh initiation into the miracle of presence.

Allow your eyelids to part very gradually. Feel the softness of the birth everywhere. Enjoy the ease and sweetness of simply resting as you are. At your own rhythm, without disturbing this feeling of quiet, support yourself into a sitting position. Sit for a while, savoring the stillness of *Savasana*.

> The law of Wonder rules my life at last
> I burn each second of my life to love
> Each second of my life burns out in love
> In each leaping second love lives afresh.
>
> —RUMI, from the *Rubaiyat*[16]

Savasana in Daily Life

As you will experience, the relaxation and peace of *Savasana* are the gateway to deep concentration, meditation, and Oneness. It takes consistent and devoted practice to keep drawing your awareness inside so that it's not excessively pulled to outer distractions, and to release the ego from its fear of drowning in the Self.

In our practice of *Savasana* we come to a precipice where we may soar beyond the mind. If we're deeply and profoundly relaxed, and grace descends, we may enter that place of pure consciousness where we experience ourselves as timeless, spacious awareness, both outside and inside time. As Iyengar masterfully describes, "The ultimate yogic triumph is to live in *kaivalya,* outside time, you might say, but really inside it, inside its heart, disconnected from past and from future. That is to live always in the kernel of the present. It is the integration of the true nature of time in consciousness, and *Savasana* is the key."[17]

This integration of time in consciousness is one of the supreme delights of the Sacred Marriage. Through experiencing this timeless, spacious awareness in *Savasana,* we can gradually learn to access it in the busyness of our daily lives, and to act and communicate from it.

As we deepen our practice of *Savasana,* we deepen our ability to return home to our true essence and divine source. As this ability to directly connect to the eternal wellspring of love and inspiration grows more firmly established, we will act from this place of peace, truth, clarity, and compassion in increasingly healing and transformative ways. Then, our experience of *Savasana,* and indeed our whole yoga practice, will reveal itself as the glowing, unshakeable foundation of our lives, and our lives will serve and benefit all beings.

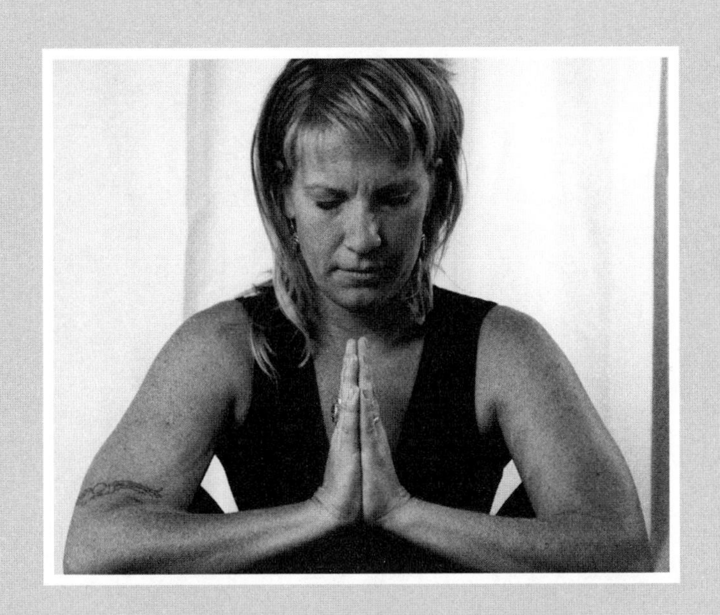

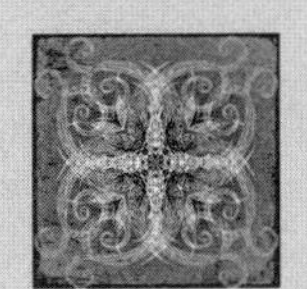 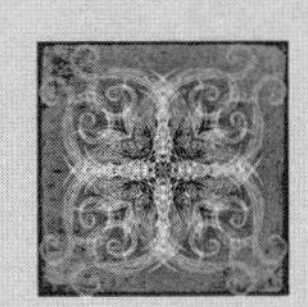 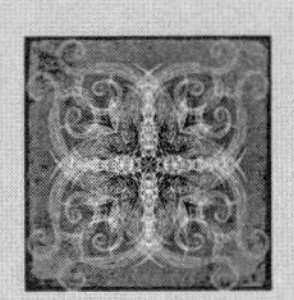

FOUR
The Joy of Transcendence

The Five Great Joys

Imagine the Sacred Marriage of all seeming dualities—Immanence and Transcendence, Feminine and Masculine, Earth and Heaven, Body and Spirit—as a vast and all-empowering sun. Five flames flare out of that sun to illumine the body, mind, heart, and spirit. Celebrating the power of these five great joys with conscious yoga practice helps to incarnate and embody the vision of the Sacred Marriage. Practiced with devotion, they engender the experience of the Sacred Marriage in the being who celebrates them. The following five chapters explore the essence of these five great joys, and offer practices for awakening and deeply experiencing them in one's entire being.

The Joy of Transcendence

The universe, the mystics of all traditions tell us, is perpetually recreated out of an infinite light-fire that is at once Being, Consciousness, and Bliss—known in Sanskrit as *Sat/Chit/Ananda.* This all-conscious, ecstatic light-fire is called by many names: Brahman in Hinduism, God in Judaism and Christianity, Allah in Islam, Shunyata (the Void) in Buddhism, and The Tao in Taoism. This is the Transcendent One, the Mother-Father, the Infinite Self, from which all universes stream, and in which all things and beings in all realms have their essential origin. On the highest levels of mystical experience, the human being who has concentrated her whole essence in the Divine enters consciously into this eternal light and knows herself to be One with its bliss and joy.

In the Upanishads the sage Uddalaka tells his son, "There is nothing that does not come from the One. The One is the Truth. The One is the Supreme Self. *Tat Tvam Asi,* You are That, You are That."[1]

As it is written in the yogic masterpiece the Ashtavakra Gita:

Yesterday
I lived bewildered,
In illusion.

But now I am awake,
Flawless and serene.
Beyond the world.

From my light
The body and world arise.

I see the infinite Self

As a wave,
Seething and foaming,
Is only water

So all creation,
Streaming out of the Self,
Is only the Self.[2]

This ancient celebration of transcendent identity is the fundamental ground of the authentic practice of yoga. One of the limitations of some modern schools of yoga is that they concentrate on the physical dimension of existence without also fully embracing the awareness that, as the Buddha said, "Form is Emptiness, Emptiness is Form." Without rooting yoga practice in the joy of transcendence, the nectar of experiencing this essential marriage between form and emptiness, matter and light, body and bliss-consciousness, individual existence and spacious eternal being cannot be tasted.

Just as exquisite stained glass remains dull until sun streams through it and awakens its colors to brilliant life, so our bodies cannot be experienced in their full mysterious vibrancy until we open to their origin in light-consciousness. And just as the music of a great composer requires the full being—body, mind, heart, and soul—of a devoted musician to be transmitted, so the practice of authentic yoga invites our full self to be present in and receptive to the radiance of origin. Then our bodies become conscious instruments of the music of the light that is the music of our innermost spirit.

The blessing of the practice of yoga, then, is that it can ground our whole being in the peace and lucid bliss of the eternal presence. It floods not only our bodies, but also our hearts and minds with direct experience of our origin in the One. It is this direct experience, beyond concept or dogma, which enables us to realize the ultimate mystery of our individual self as a hologram of the entire universe.

Yoga Practice Sequence to Celebrate the Joy of Transcendence

- Child's Pose – *Adho Mukha Virasana*
- Hands and Knees Pose
- Downward-facing Dog Pose – *Adho Mukha Svanasana*
- Lunge Pose
- Mountain Pose – *Tadanasa*
- Sun Salutations – *Surya Namaskar*
- Warrior Pose I – *Virbhadrasana I*
- Warrior Pose II – *Virbhadrasana II*
- Hero Pose – *Virasana*
- Seated Twist – *Bharadvajasana*
- One-legged Sitting Forward Bend – *Janu Sirsasana*
- Seated Forward Bend – *Paschimottanasana*
- Reclined Bound Angle Pose – *Supta Baddha Konasana*
- Calves Elevated on Chair or Pillows
- Corpse Pose – *Savasana*

Behold the body, born of dust, how perfect it has become,
Why should you fear its end?
When were you ever made less by dying?
When you pass beyond this human form,
No doubt you will become an angel and soar through the heavens,
But don't stop there, even heavenly bodies grow old,
Pass again from the heavenly realm and
Plunge, plunge into the vast ocean of consciousness,
Let the drop of water that is you become a hundred mighty seas.
But do not think that the drop alone becomes the ocean.
The ocean, too, becomes the drop.

—RUMI[3]

The following yoga poses celebrate and initiate you into the great joy of transcendence. They will enable you to embody the vivid, blissful light-energy of your true nature, serving as a pathway to awaken your body and mind to the dynamic dance of this divine light-energy.

Begin by lighting a candle to clarify your focus and connect you with your deepest intention. As you gaze at the candle, imagine the power and pure beauty of this light permeating and illumining every cell in your body. Pray to become the light embodied, a flame of divine love that burns with calm sacred passion.

Place before the sun a burning candle
And watch its brilliance disappear before that blaze
The candle exists no longer
But is transformed into the Light.

—RUMI[4]

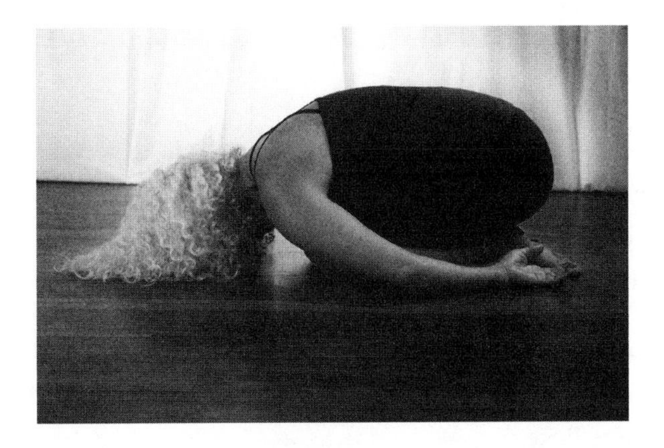

Child's Pose
Adho Mukha Virasana

We begin our practice of the great joy of transcendence with Child's Pose, because all the mystical traditions agree that it is through the humility, innocence, trust, and surrender of child-mind that we can gracefully enter the transcendent. To embody the light is to be born as a divine child, birthed from the union of all seeming dualities: masculine and feminine, transcendent and immanent, light and dark, spirit and body.

Sit back on your heels, your knees slightly apart. Gradually bend forward, using your hands for support. Place your forehead on your mat or a bolster, gently placing your hands back by your feet. Your body is now softly curling; your back widening.

Bring your awareness fully into your breath, and notice how in this position the breath naturally flows to the back of your lungs, opening the back ribs like spreading feathers. As your back ribs become suppler, feel your kidneys widening like wings, and the skin of your back unraveling.

Rumi wrote, "How can you ever hope to know the Beloved, without becoming in every cell, the lover?" Imagine every cell awakening and becoming the lover, igniting millions of soft fires in your body-mind. Allow the warm glow of these fires to illuminate your entire being.

While keeping your focus on the light of the inner fires, slowly and tenderly lengthen your arms out in front of you. Bring your awareness to your breath, and let it wash over you again and again, returning you to the root of yourself.

> You may think that you are earthly beings but you have been kneaded from the substance of certainty. You are the guardians of God's light, so come, return to the root of the root of your own self.
>
> —RUMI[5]

Imagine yourself like an ember, aglow with golden light.

Hands and Knees Pose

Slowly move to your hands and knees, feeling them supported by the earth. Gaze at your hands as if you've never seen hands before. Marvel at their intricacy and mystery. Feel the sun at the center of your palms, and see your fingers as its radiating rays. Become aware of that strong, solar energy streaming up your hands, through your arms, into your heart, belly, and pelvis, and down your legs into your feet.

Inhale, lifting your tailbone and head, and feel your spine undulating through the core of your body like seaweed moving in a wave, releasing the front of your spine. As you exhale, draw your tailbone and head downward and arch your spine upward, the back of your spine now rippling open.

Continue this rocking movement, feeling how centering it is to synchronize the wave of your spine with the wave of your breath. Explore moving your hips to the sides, and in circles. Release into your own rhythm—body, mind, and breath uniting.

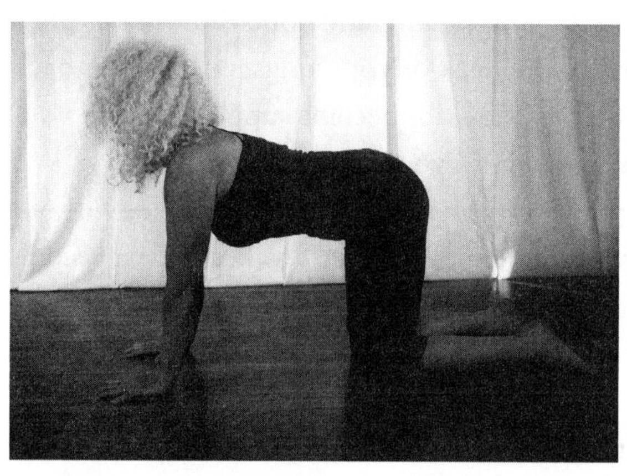

Immerse your mind in this sensuous snake-like movement of your spine. Enjoy the sacred dance of your spine, hips, shoulders, and breath.

Downward-facing Dog Pose
Adho Mukha Svanasana
From the Hands and Knees Pose, curl your toes under. Exhale, and as if your belly were a helium balloon, let it lift your hips up to the sky, elongating your spine and lengthening your legs from hips to heels, coming into the Downward-facing Dog Pose. If your back or legs hurt, keep your knees bent.

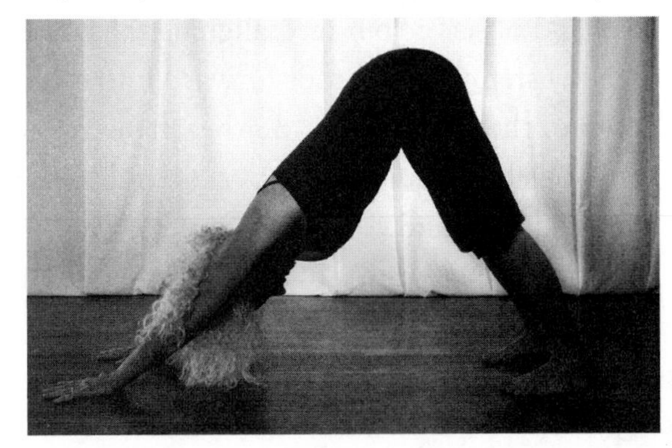

Embed your hands and feet into the earth, imagining them sinking into warm mud, while your tailbone softly floats. Let your head drop, pouring all lingering thoughts like water onto the earth, quieting your mind. Feel the base of your skull loosen, and your neck soften.

Explore arching your back into a backbend like a dog bowing, or rounding your back into a forward bend like a cat. Be playful, and gentle, never forcing anything. If you become tired, rest in Child's Pose (See page 51), returning to Downward-facing Dog Pose when you feel ready. Experiment with how your body wants to move. Step from foot to foot, bend your knees, or come up onto your toes. Let the joy and delight of exploration sparkle throughout every cell of your body.

Lunge Pose
From Dog Pose, come into Lunge Pose by stepping your right foot forward between your hands, aligning your right knee over your right ankle, and releasing your left knee, shin, and the top of your foot to the floor. Lift your arms overhead, opening to the light above. Let your heart soar like an eagle, while your feet continue to send roots into the earth. Soften your eyes. Stay for a few breaths.

From Lunge Pose, step your right foot back and return to Dog Pose.

Lengthen your body evenly, and as you elongate, relish the joy of release. Feel your body smiling as it becomes free. Lift your head and look at your hands, enlivening them. Point your middle fingers straight ahead. Drop your head and observe your feet, aligning them evenly.

Now step your left foot forward into a lunge, releasing your right knee down to the floor. From your heart, sweep your arms up. Keep your eyes soft, your brain quiet, and your face relaxed. Feel your feet and legs stable and grounded, and your pelvis watery, waving and lifting with your breath. Experience the airiness of your heart, and the spacious emptiness of your head.

To come out of the pose, step your right foot toward your hands, bending your knees and dropping your head, and rest in the Standing Forward Bend Pose (See page 103). Exhale, and slowly roll up to standing.

Mountain Pose
Tadasana

Mountain Pose, *Tadasana,* enables you to incarnate the fully grounded majesty of your human divinity. In *Tadasana,* you align yourself with the luminous steadiness and grandeur of the mountain.

Feel your feet on earth, your heart warm and glowing. Allow your body to find its natural skeletal alignment, bones resting evenly on bones so that your muscles don't overwork to create balance.

Become aware of the exquisite and intricate architecture of your body standing. Relax your hands, releasing whatever you're holding, and feel the quiet ecstasy of letting go. Notice the vibrant, pulsing connection of your hands and feet with the earth, and allow Mountain Pose to help you to stand simply in the pure and naked presence of this moment. (See page 39 in Chapter Three, "The Sacred Marriage Yoga Practice," for more detailed instructions on this pose.)

Without judgment, watch how you stand and how you feel.

Krishnamurti said that observation without judgment is the highest form of spiritual practice. Thoughts and emotions will come and go. Releasing evaluation or attachment, allow them to pass over you like clouds drifting across a mountain.

In Taoism, our original nature is described as being like an "uncarved rock." Be that uncarved rock. Sound a silent *OM*, in the depths of your heart, and experience your heart opening like a vast light-flower in the core of your body, the fire at the center of the mountain. "The heart," as Rumi tells us in the *Mathnawi*, "is nothing but the Sea of Light . . . the place of the vision of God.'"[6]

> In the Ocean of the Heart love opens its mouth
> And gulps down the two worlds like a whale.
>
> Understand what cannot be understood!
> Hear from the heart wordless mysteries!
> In our stone-dark hearts there burns a fire
> That burns all veils to their root and foundation.
> When the veils have been burned away
> Then the heart will understand completely.
> Ancient Love will unfold ever-fresh forms
> In the heart of the Spirit, in the core of the heart.
>
> —RUMI[7]

Sun Salutations

Surya Namaskar

Uniting transcendence and immanence, the Sun Salutation invokes the all-transforming light-energy of the sun. This Shakti energy awakens our subtle energy centers and illuminates every cell. By practicing Sun Salutation as a profound prayer, we unveil the embodied suns that we are and experience the holy joy of living as the Light.

We receive the solar energy into our bodies with each inhalation, and with each exhalation offer it back to the Source. As embodied suns, we worship our Mother-Father, the great Sun. When we practice with this consciousness, gratitude and bliss suffuse our whole being.

Sun Salutation: Drawing Down the Light

Begin in Mountain Pose *(Tadasana)* by imagining yourself surrounded by a circle of golden light, and visualize your heart as a softly pulsing sun. This enables you to consciously enter your mystical light-body. When your visualization is strong and vivid, tenderly and with devotion, draw your hands together in front of your heart center, feeling its radiant warmth.

Pressing the roots of your thumbs into your heart center, feel your heart pulsing with light-energy. Bow your head slightly, so that it rests in the soft, warm, luminous bed of your heart.

Open your hands from your heart center, releasing your arms down to your sides, palms turned out. Feel your arms and hands extend from the core of your heart. Become aware of the vibrant line of energy streaming from the heart sun, through your shoulders and down your arms into the glow of your fingertips.

Let your arms slowly rise like wings spreading from your heart center. Experience the light radiating from you, and with your hands draw that circle of golden light around you. As your hands gradually come together, feel your left and right sides uniting as one. Sense how your fingertips flare upwards from the sun of your heart, your belly, and your feet.

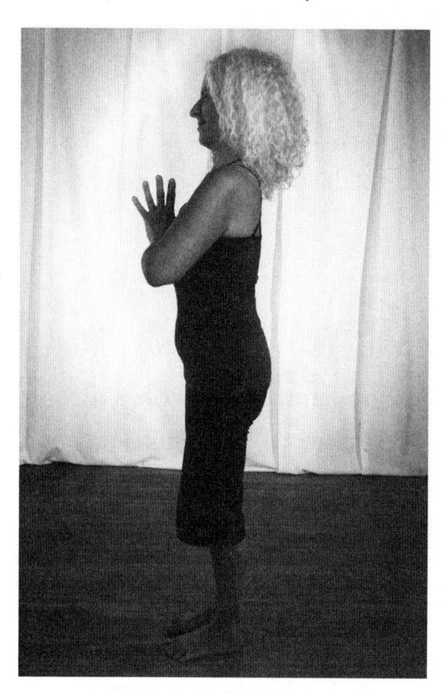

Empowered by the light-energy you have invoked, now gratefully draw down that divine radiance into the core of your body and awaken your sacred centers.

Very slowly lowering your joined palms, pull the transcendent light down through the crown of your head. As you do so, visualize the crown chakra opening like a thousand-petaled lotus of diamond light.

Continue slowly drawing down the light through the third eye, awakening and visualizing it as a diamond, streaming light in all directions and radiating its crystalline clarity everywhere.

Continuing down through the center of your throat, visualize that center opening like a rich red rose, illumined from within by soft golden light.

Bring your hands to rest in front of your heart, visualizing your heart center like a burning golden chalice, glowing with light.

Feel the simplicity of standing with your feet rooted on earth, and the crown of your head open to the light above. The sacred energies of earth and heaven meet and merge now in the marriage bed of your heart.

Simple Sun Salutation

Once again, empty your hands and sweep your arms out, letting the golden wings of your heart open.

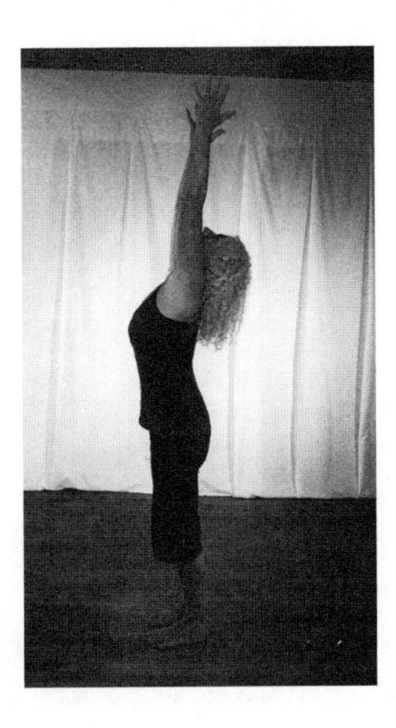

Join your hands above you, and then open them out to the sides, sweeping your arms down from your heart as you bow forward. Hinge deeply from the hip joints, bending your knees if that is more comfortable for you. Release your hands to the earth, and touch it with reverence.

Slowly slide one foot back and then the other, balancing in the Plank Pose, like a high push-up position.

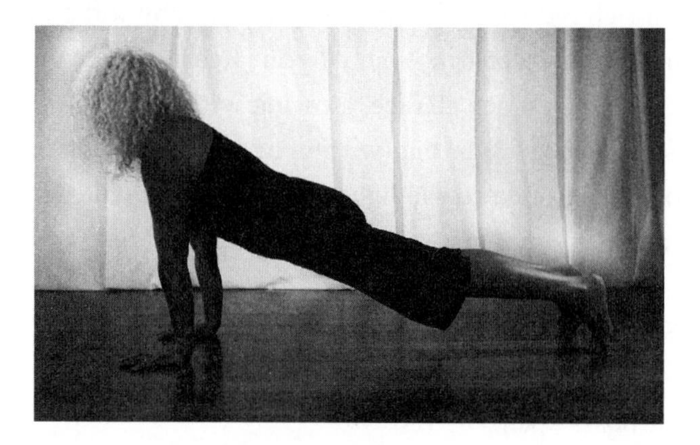

From Plank Pose, you can either: release your knees, chest, and chin to the floor, then lift your heart up, like the sun rising, its rays illuminating the sky, into a simple Cobra Pose (See page 106); or if you have the strength, release down into a low push-up position, then straighten your arms, lifting your heart up.

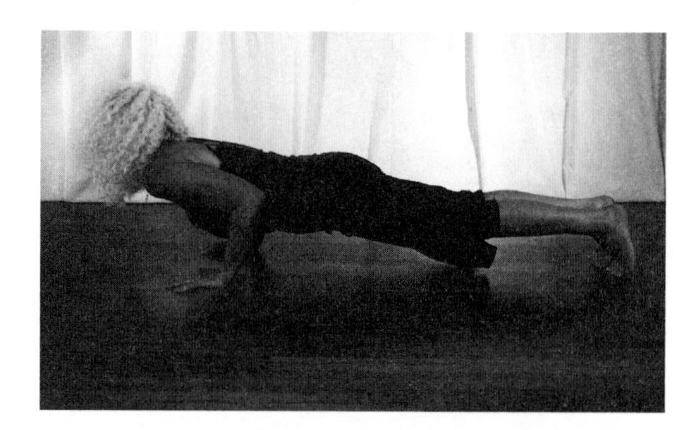

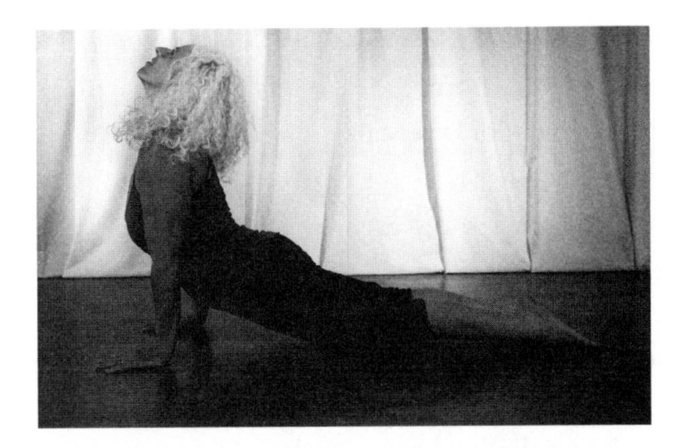

From Cobra or Upward-facing Dog Pose, either rest in Child's Pose or go directly into Downward-facing Dog Pose.

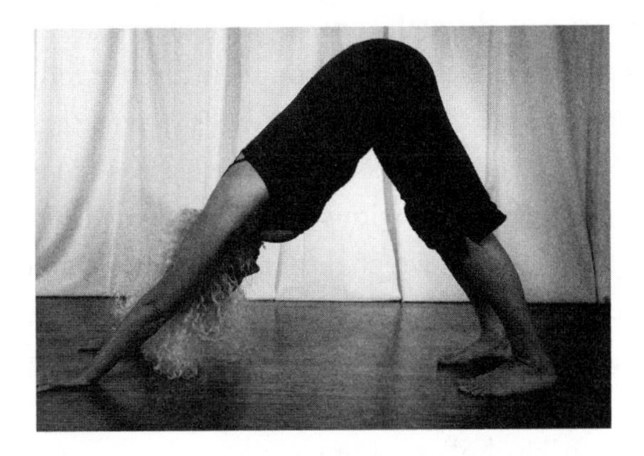

From Dog Pose, bend your knees and lengthen back into the total surrender of Child's Pose. Release your forehead onto the floor, softening your eyes, quieting your mind, and resting on the earth.

The brilliant sun that shines in every heart
For the heaven's earth and all creatures
What a blessing!
The heart can't wait to speak of this ecstasy
The soul is kissing the earth, saying
Oh God, what a blessing!

Fill me with the wine of your silence,
Let it soak my every pore
For the inner splendor it reveals
Is a blessing
Is a blessing.
—RUMI[8]

Feel the blessing of your body kissing the earth.

Now slowly sweep forward again to your hands and knees. Curl your toes under; lift your belly, and come back to Downward-facing Dog Pose. Step one foot forward between your hands, again coming into a lunge, and then bring the other foot forward, returning to the Standing Forward Bend. Bend your knees, rise up through your belly and heart, and sweep your arms out to the sides and over the head, as you float up to standing. Lifting your heart, keep your eyes soft as they gaze upwards into the light. Your feet are firmly on earth, while your heart opens to the transcendent.

Again draw the light down with your palms joined, through the thousand-petaled lotus of the crown chakra, through the diamond light of the third eye, through the rich red rose of the throat, into the luminous golden chalice of the heart. Arrive back in the heart center, with gratitude and wonder. Remember, throughout, that this practice of honoring and embodying the divine light is one of the holiest of prayers.

Creating Your Own Sun Salutation

Now let your body explore whatever form of Sun Salutation your intuition suggests to you. At your own rhythm, find your unique way of moving prayerfully through each cycle, practicing at least five or six cycles, to allow the repetition of the movement to quiet your mind and deepen your experience of embodying the light.

Explore variations of Sun Salutation, moving at your own rhythm and following your breath. Trust and honor your way of greeting the light.

You can start with very simple Sun Salutations to warm up, maybe simply stepping back from the Standing Forward Bend to Dog Pose, and then back to the Forward Bend and up again. Rest in Child's Pose at any time.

More experienced students will enjoy adding any of the standing poses, or any asanas, into the flow of the Sun Salutation. Let your intuition guide you in a graceful flow from pose to pose. For example, try adding Warrior I or II.

Warrior I
Virbhadrasana I

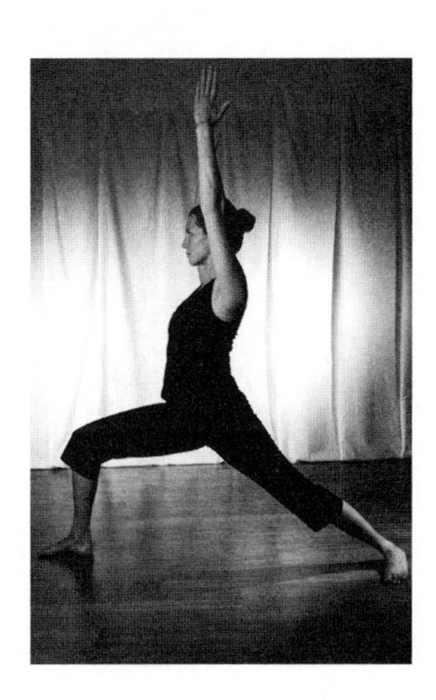

From Dog Pose, step your right foot forward into a high lunge. Turning the left foot into a 45-degree angle, rotate your hips to face the short end of your mat. Press down through your right foot, and from your heart sweep your arms over your head, coming into Warrior I. Stay for three to five breaths, lifting through your pelvic floor, while scooping your belly toward the back of the diaphragm. Allow that lifting energy to surge up into the sun of your heart. Either return to Dog Pose, or move to Warrior II.

Warrior II
Virbhadrasana II

From Warrior I, inhale, and keeping your heart radiating in all directions, rotate your torso to face the long end of your mat, while spreading your

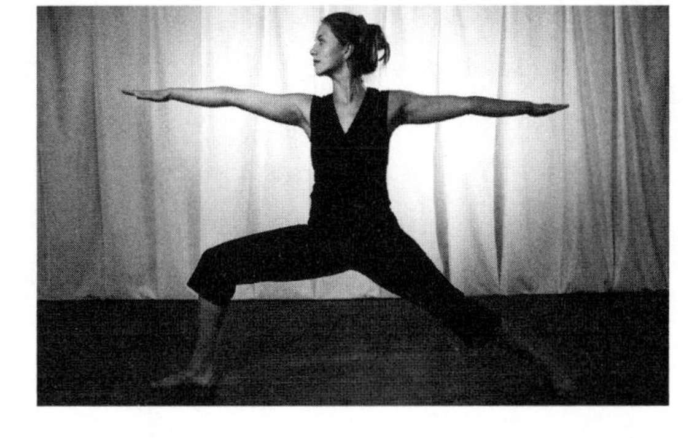

arms out until they're parallel to the floor. Balance over the midline of your body, poised in the present moment between past and future. Turn your head and gaze over your right hand. Stay for three to five breaths, and then sweep your arms overhead like wings opening, and turn your feet and release down into Warrior I to the left side. After three to five breaths, spread out to Warrior II on the left, then come down to Dog Pose and continue your Sun Salutation sequence.

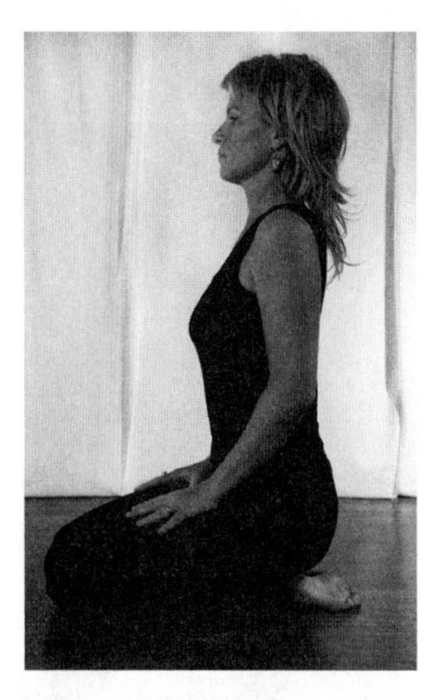

Hero Pose
Virasana
Sit back on your heels, or sit on a block or blankets. Your feet are on either side of your hips, pointing straight back to protect your knee joints from injury. If you experience knee pain in this pose, consult an experienced yoga teacher on how to use props to create comfort. If you feel ankle or foot pain, try blankets underneath your legs and feet.

Rest your hands on your thighs. Root your legs down into the earth, and feel your spine rising, your heart ascending, and the crown of your head opening to receive the light. You may interlock your fingers and lift your arms over your head, reaching toward the transcendent. Stay five to ten breaths, aligning the core channel of your body, and noticing how the life energy (prana) rises up through the cylinder of your torso.

Seated Twist
Bharadvajasana
From the Hero Pose, shift your legs to the left, placing your feet next to your left hip, and resting the top of your right foot on the arch of the left foot. Awaken your feet, drawing energy up the legs into your pelvis. Scoop up through your belly, lifting your heart. You can place a small support under your right sitting bone to keep your pelvis level.

Inhale, and lengthen from your tailbone to the crown of your head. Exhale, and begin releasing your belly toward the right, continuing to root your feet

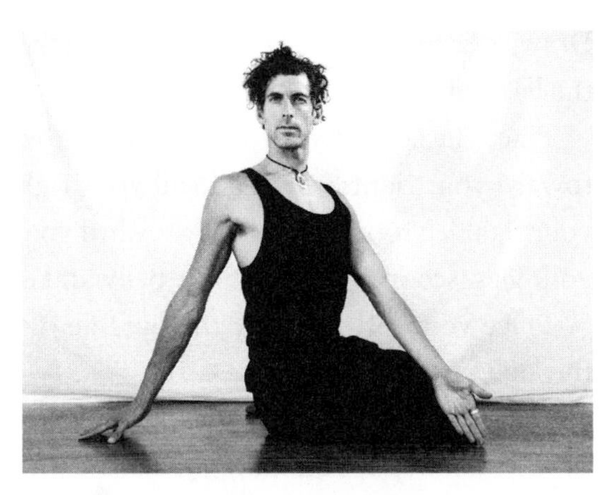

and legs into the floor. Root, rise, and release with each breath. With each exhalation, gradually turn from your belly, ribs, and shoulders, allowing your neck and head to gently receive the twist, rather than leading the twist.

Place your right hand behind you and move down into the earth through your fingers. Rest your left hand lightly on the outside of your right thigh. Move back, through your left thigh and forward from the right hip to right knee, widening the thighs slightly apart, like blades of scissors opening.

Feel the energy spiraling up your spine, and open the crown of your head to the descending light bathing you like a gentle shower. Stay three to five breaths then slowly return to center, resting for a few breaths in Hero Pose before releasing to the other side. After completing the other side, release your legs straight out in front of you for a few breaths.

Sitting Forward Bend
Janu Sirsasana

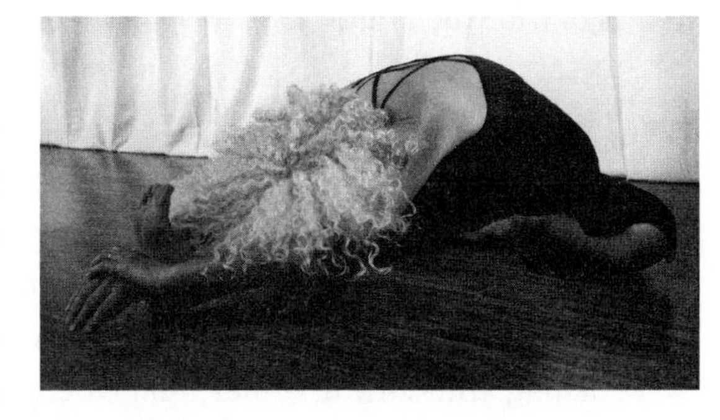

Please consult a health professional before practicing this pose if you have a knee or back injury.

Sit with your legs outstretched, opening the backs of your legs evenly onto the floor. If your pelvis feels like it's tipping backward, sit on a folded blanket for support.

Draw your right foot toward you and put the fingers of your right hand between your thigh and calf muscles as you let your knee roll to the outside.

Draw your fingers out slowly, separating the thigh and calf muscles to soften the back of the knee.

Place the sole of your right foot on the inside of your left thigh. Turn toward your right knee, and roll your right thigh to the outside. Keeping your right leg rooted, turn back toward your left leg. Moving down through your legs, scoop up through the belly and elongate your spine.

Place your left hand by the outside of your left hip, and move down through your hand into the earth. Place your right hand on the outside of your left leg, and gently turn to face that leg. Hinging deep in the hip joints, rather than overly rounding the back, slowly lengthen your torso over the inside of your left leg.

Hold your left leg or foot with both hands, or put a strap around the foot, consciously releasing forward with each breath, rather than pulling yourself over. Inhale, and elongate your spine. Exhale, and lifting your belly, soften over your legs. Allow your forehead to rest on a support. You may wish to draw a bolster up under the entire torso to support the front of your spine, letting it round evenly as you release forward.

Notice your back widening and your mind quieting in this gentle forward bend. As you drop deeply inside yourself, consciously draw in the surrounding light you've felt around you in your practice. Open to the light inside as well as outside the body.

Seated Forward Bend

Paschimottanasana

Sit with your legs outstretched, your feet active, and your hips slightly elevated on a folded blanket. Spread the backs of your legs into the floor, and elongate your spine upwards, lifting the chest.

Widening your sitting bones, hinge deeply in your groin, and slowly begin to soften forward. You can put a strap around your feet, or place your hands on your legs or feet, wherever they naturally reach. Elongate your spine with each inhalation, and soften and surrender your spine with each exhalation. As you fold forward into yourself, evenly round your

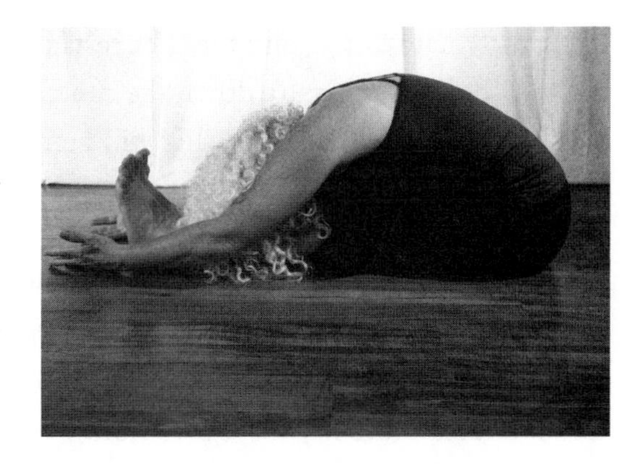

spine into a crescent moon, reflecting the light of the sun.

Rest your head on a bolster, and drop inward. In the quiet of your resting body, listen to the whisperings of your heart. Gaze with your inner eyes at the light within you, seeing the brightness of your inner body.

> We search for Him here and there, while looking right at Him.
> Sitting by his side, we ask: Oh Beloved, where is the Beloved?
> Enough with such questions
> Let silence take you to the core of life.
> All your talk is worthless when compared with one whisper of the Beloved.
>
> —RUMI[9]

Rest here at least five breaths, then on an exhalation, lift your belly and slowly roll up to sitting.

Reclined Bound Angle Pose
Supta Baddha Konasana

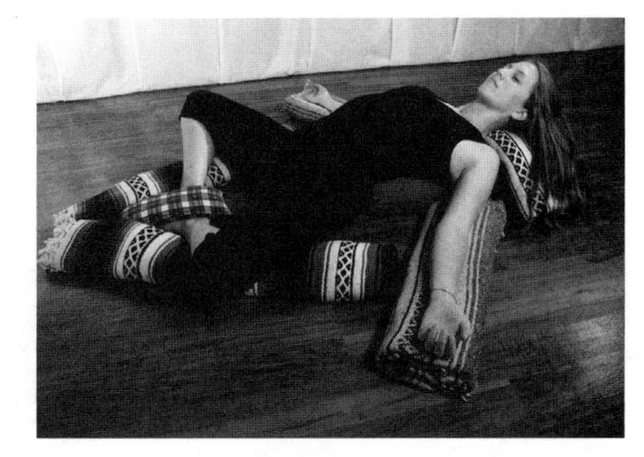

This pose creates a sense of deep relaxation. The fully supported body can completely release, and the mind can transcend the usual boundaries of personality. Beliefs, stories, and opinions melt away. The thought-waves of the mind resolve back into their source, and the Seer rests in the Self (Yoga Sutras I-2, I-3).[10]

Put a bolster vertically down the center of your mat, and place a folded blanket on the far end of it (this will be for your neck and head). Roll up two blankets and put them on either sides of the near end of your mat (these will go under your thighs). You can also place two rolled-up blankets on either side of the bolster to support your arms, or use pillows.

Sit facing away from the bolster, drawing it up to your tailbone. Bring the soles of your feet together. You can roll a blanket and place it over the feet and tuck it under your legs to hold your feet together. Open your knees out to the sides, and let your thighs rest on the rolled blankets.

Lengthen your back down onto the bolster, placing your neck and head on the folded blanket. Adjust your props so that your forehead is higher than your chin; your chin higher than your chest; and your chest higher than your belly. Place an eye pillow over your eyes, and rest your arms on the center of the rolled blankets.

Sink back into your supports, allowing yourself to be held like a small child in its mother's arms. Watch the natural rhythm of your breath, and notice how as you relax your breath grows softer and slower. Feel your body and mind rocked in the cradle of your breath. Relax as long as you like. When you're ready to come out of the pose, draw your knees together and lengthen your legs out, resting back on your bolster for a few more breaths. Then roll to the right side, enjoying the sweetness of resting on earth.

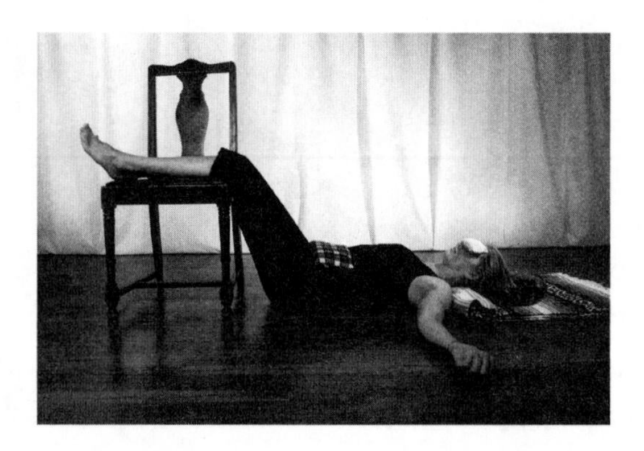

Calves Elevated on Chair or Pillows

Gather some pillows or bolsters and place them under your calves, resting on your back. Or draw a chair close to your body and rest your legs on its seat. Place an eye pillow over your eyes and release your arms to the sides, palms up.

> The whole world could be choked with thorns:
> A lover's heart will stay a rose garden.
> The wheel of heaven could wind to a halt:
> The world of lovers will go on turning.
> Even if every being grew sad, a lover's soul
> Will still stay fresh, vibrant, light.
> Are all the candles out? Hand them to a lover—
> A lover shoots out a hundred thousand fires.
> —RUMI[11]

Corpse Pose
Savasana

Since we have already unfolded the richness and majesty of *Savasana* in detail in the Yoga Practice to Celebrate the Sacred Marriage (Chapter Three), from now on all descriptions of *Savasana* will focus on instructions relevant to the focus of each chapter. You may want to refresh your memory by referring to the detailed instructions for *Savasana* in Chapter Three.

In this *Savasana* celebrating transcendence, the practice focuses on opening the entire bodymind to the transcendent light. Sit on your mat with your knees up and your feet flat. Release back to your elbows,

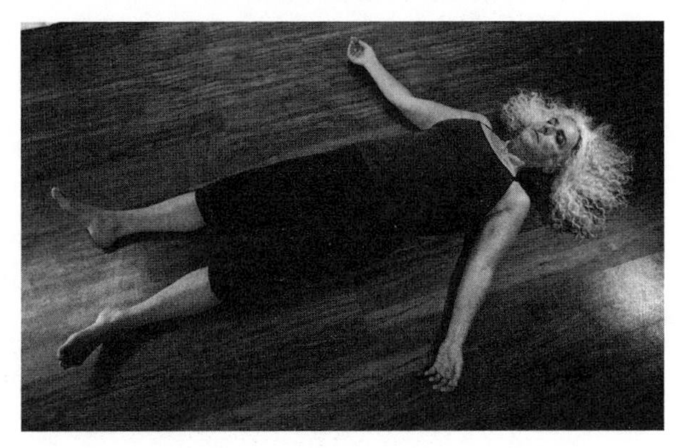

and pause to let your belly soften. Feel your kidneys release and the back of your waist lengthen. Elongate your spine as you rest back onto the floor. Place an eye pillow over your eyes. Extend your arms out to the sides, turning your palms upwards; your hands are soft like babies' hands. Feel your back body widening, and your front body releasing back into its embrace.

Simply notice the natural inclination of your body to release back into the earth, like water flowing downhill or snow melting in the warmth of the sun. Release into the cauldron of the earth beneath you. Just as a child would snuggle back into its mother's arms, find the comfort of being able to lie back and let go. The boundaries of your body soften and begin to dissolve.

When thoughts arise, let them float downstream. Focus on your breath gently flowing through your body like a wave, washing through you. As you notice your body beginning to relax and settle back into the silence, observe also the gradual settling of the mind. As Patanjali explains in the Yoga Sutras (I-2), yoga is this dissolving of the thought waves of the mind back into the source.

Your skin becomes more porous and transparent, almost translucent, so that the light of your innermost self radiates out from you in all directions, and the light surrounding you permeates your body from all sides, turning you into a brilliant lamp.

> The lamps are different
> But the Light is the same.
> So many garish lamps in the dying brain's lamp shop
> Forget about them.
> Concentrate on essence, concentrate on Light.
> In lucid bliss, calmly smoking off its own holy fire
> The light streams toward you from all things,
> All people, all possible permutations of good, evil, thought, passion.
> The lamps are different
> But the Light is the same.

One matter, one energy, one Light, one Light-mind,
Endlessly emanating all things.
One turning and burning diamond.
One, one, one.
Ground yourself, strip yourself down,
To blind loving silence.
Stay there, until you see
You are gazing at the Light
with its own ageless eyes.

—RUMI[12]

In this *Savasana* of the transcendent, visualize bathing yourself in waves of divine light. Consciously breathe this diamond light in and out. See the diamond light constantly descending in blessing, and offer yourself up to it in prayer and gratitude. With each inhalation, absorb the light freely, and with each exhalation, effortlessly radiate it out as an offering to all beings.

Now slowly, from the spaciousness of *Savasana,* gently draw your awareness to your breath. With the body so relaxed and receptive, notice how freely the breath flows. The doors and the windows of the body are open, so that the exquisite cooling and cleansing light-winds of the breath can wash through and renew you.

Allow these winds of breath to awaken your body-mind, bathing each cell in the dawn light of renewal. Feel the subtle transformation on the minutest molecular level that this immersion in the light-energy awakens in your body.

When you feel ready, move from the position of the corpse *(Savasana).* Roll onto your right side, into the position of the embryo—of birth—feeling the support of the whole earth beneath you as you turn. Feel that you are being birthed in every cell of your body as a divine/human being—the divine child. Rest on Mother Earth, the way a baby rests on its mother's body. Feel the tenderness of her support and the surrender of your being to her, as she awakens you to ever greater and more luminous depths of yourself.

> Awake awhile.
>
> It does not have to be forever.
> Right now.
>
> One step upon the Sky's soft skirt would be enough.
>
> Awake awhile.
> Just one True moment of Love will last for days.
>
> Rest all your elaborate plans and tactics for knowing Him,
> For they are all just frozen spring buds
> Far, so far from Summer's Divine Gold.
>
> Awake, my dear.
> Be kind to your sleeping heart.
> Take it out into the vast fields of Light
> And let it breathe.
>
> Say, "Love, give me back my wings.
> Lift me, lift me nearer."
>
> Say to the sun and moon, say to our dear Friend,
>
> I will take You up now, Beloved,
> On that wonderful dance You promised!
>
> —HAFIZ[13]

That wonderful dance the Beloved promised is now alive in every cell of your being. At your own rhythm, when you feel like moving, slowly support yourself up to a sitting position. Sit as the divine radiant human being that you are, in all your beauty, majesty, and dignity.

Namaste.

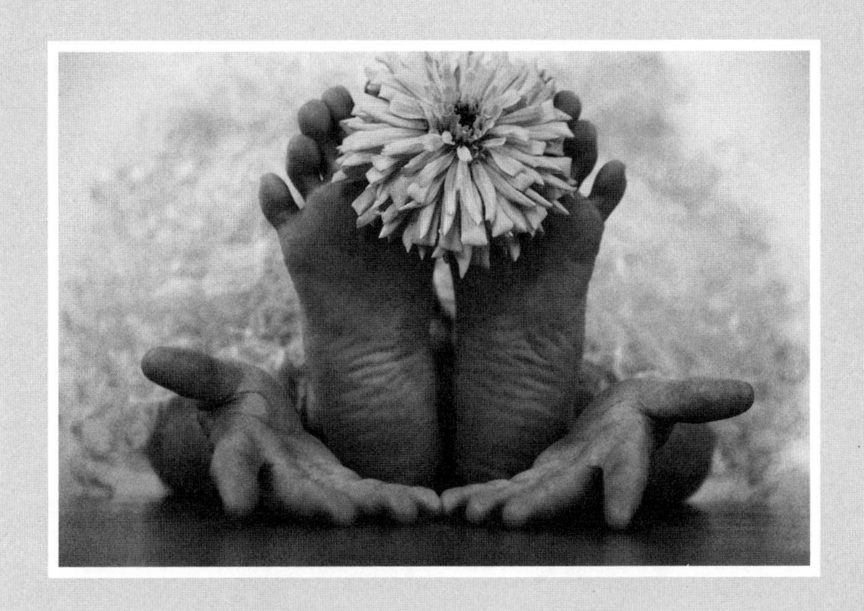

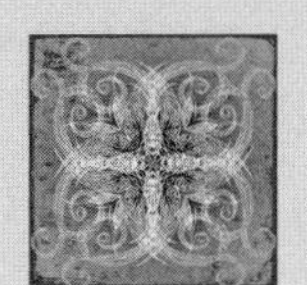 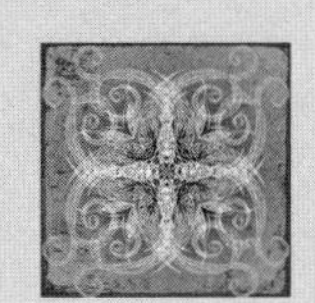 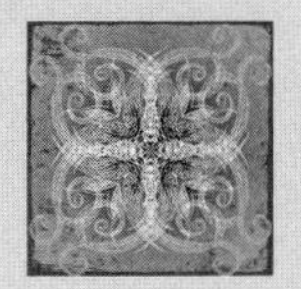

FIVE
The Joy of Creation

Smile, O voluptuous cool-breath'd earth!
Earth of the slumbering and liquid trees!
Earth of departed sunset—earth of the mountains misty-topt!
Earth of the vitreous pour of the full moon just tinged with blue!
Earth of shine and dark mottling the tide of the river!
Earth of the limpid gray of clouds brighter and clearer for my sake!
Far-swooping elbow'd earth—rich apple-blossom'd earth!
Smile—for your lover comes.
Prodigal, you have given me love—
Therefore I to you give love!
O unspeakable passionate love.

—WALT WHITMAN[1]

Love the earth and sun and animals ... dismiss whatever insults your own soul, and your very flesh shall be a great poem and have the richest fluency not only in its words but in the silent lines of its lips and face and between the lashes of your eyes and in every motion of your body.

—WALT WHITMAN[2]

For those who have awakened in every tradition, the Creation reveals itself as the manifested glory of the Sacred Feminine. Each leaf, each stone, each leaping dolphin, each incandescent fish, each gazelle, each mountain, each river, are all different expressions of the one eternal Mother, children of Her light-womb.

Rumi wrote, "Adore and love the Beloved, with your whole being, and the Beloved will reveal to you that each thing in the universe is a vessel full to the brim with wisdom and beauty. The Beloved will show you that each thing is one drop from the boundless river of infinite beauty."[3] There was a Moroccan Sufi master from Fez so attuned to the sacred splendor of each created thing that the sight of one open rose would send him into ecstasy for a day. His disciples, impatient with his trances, would only allow him to look at a flower after six o'clock in the evening. When he died, they placed one solitary red rose on his tomb and it is said that it turned to gold.

To be awake is to revere, cherish, and recognize each created thing and the creation itself as different facets of the transcendent diamond of the One. As Allah announces in one of the Prophet Muhammad's sacred sayings: "I was a hidden treasure and wanted to be known. That is why I created the world."

Heart Yoga was matured and distilled in the Kootenay Mountains of British Columbia. The snow-capped peaks that surrounded the small sanctuary where we worked calmed and steadied us, and spoke to us with piercing, silent eloquence of the majesty of the Infinite Self. The vast brilliant lake at their feet turned into a molten mirror of the light of the One. The tall noble enduring firs, with their tops soaring into limitless sky and their roots intertwining in the dark earth mysteries of the forest floor, initiated us into the primordial meaning of Tree Pose. The winds, flowing down from the mountain glaciers, attuned our breathing to that breath of the Beloved that shimmers and animates each blade of grass, each running stream, each cascade of moss, each jagged rock gleaming from afternoon snows. We felt directly the company and inspiration of the ancient Vedic sages who created yoga in surroundings of similar glory. We understood, beyond thought, how the grandeur of creation birthed in the ancient yogis an answering vision of the potential grandeur of the divine human. As Rumi wrote, "Transform my heart to a placeless place of safety. Carry it to the mountains where it dies into you."[4]

We discovered for ourselves that when, as Rumi says, the heart "dies into you," the creation becomes a constant epiphany of miracle. Moses Cordovero, a Kabbalist of the sixteenth century, wrote of this awakening: "An epiphany enables you to sense creation not as something completed, but as constantly becoming, evolving, ascending. This transports you from a place where there is nothing new to a place where there is nothing old, where everything renews itself, where heaven and earth rejoice as at the moment of Creation."[5]

Our Heart Yoga of the Joy of Creation is designed to birth you into this eternal moment and this rejoicing.

A great nineteenth-century Bengali mystic, Fikirchand, sang of this manifested beauty of the transcendent One.

> My soul cries out,
> snared by the beauty
> of the formless one.
> As I cry by myself,
> night and day,
> beauty amassed before my eyes
> surpasses numberless moons and stars.
> If I look at the clouds in the sky,
> I see His beauty afloat;
> and I see Him walk on the stars
> blazing my heart.[6]

The Heart Yoga of the Joy of Creation invites us into the luminous depths of such a sacramental vision of reality, helping us see, know, and experience the entire creation as a flowering of the infinite Self that we are. From such direct sight, knowledge, and experience flows naturally a burning desire to honor, preserve, and protection Creation. Such a desire is the reward of the yoga and the oxygen of our survival now, as a frenzy of selfishness and greed threatens both our own existence and that of nature.

As we deepen our practice of the yoga of the celebration of creation, the infinite beauty that creates all beauty starts to remake us, in our psyches and bodies. We mirror increasingly in our inner and outer being that alchemy of the Sacred Feminine that is at work everywhere in the world around us. The "unspeakable passionate love" that Whitman celebrates slowly becomes the fundamental truth of our nature, and the ground of all the actions we take in and for the Creation. Our very flesh starts to become, in Whitman's words, "a great poem."

Yoga Practice Sequence to Celebrate the Joy of Creation

- Child's Pose – *Adho Mukha Virasana*
- Cat/Cow Pose
- Downward-facing Dog Pose – *Adho Mukha Svanasana*
- Mountain Pose – *Tadasana*
- Tree Pose – *Vrksasana*
- Triangle Pose – *Trikonasana*
- Standing Forward Bend – *Uttanasana*
- Eagle Pose – *Garudasana*
- Sun Salutations – *Surya Namaskar*
- Squatting Pose – *Malasana*
- Sphinx Pose – *Bhujangasana* modification
- Cobra Pose – *Bhujangasana*
- Downward-facing Dog Pose – *Adho Mukha Svanasana*
- Cross-legged Sitting – *Sukhasana*
- Corpse Pose – *Savasana*

In this section we will practice poses that celebrate the great joy of creation, the healing ecstasy that arises when we experience our identity with all beings and realize that we and all creation are a manifestation of the divine.

At this time in history when the entire creation is menaced by our ignorance of its divine origin and by our greed, the simple, direct revelations that these poses bring can transform our lives and our actions. They inspire us to become protectors and guardians, not destroyers, of our world.

We have chosen earthy and grounded asanas for this practice to enable us to feel our interconnection and interdependence with all life. They are poses that ancient yogis evolved to assume various shapes of nature, and so to experience our oneness with the natural world. Practicing these poses reveals to us this all-healing and all-empowering Oneness. It fills us with both the sacred peace and the sacred passion that endlessly dance together to create the world. These poses "teach us, and show us the way."

We call upon the earth, our planet home, with its beautiful depths and soaring
heights, its vitality and abundance of life, and together we ask that it

Teach us, and show us the Way.

We call upon the mountains, the Cascades and the Olympics, the high green
valleys and meadows filled with wild flowers, the snows that never melt, the
summits of intense silence, and we ask that they

Teach us, and show us the Way.

We call upon the waters that rim the earth, horizon to horizon, that flow in our
rivers and streams, that fall upon our gardens and fields and we ask that they

Teach us, and show us the Way.

We call upon the land which grows our food, the nurturing soil, the fertile fields,
the abundant gardens and orchards, and we ask that they

Teach us, and show us the Way.

We call upon the forest, the great trees reaching strongly to the sky with earth in
their roots and the heavens in their branches, the fir and the pine and the
cedar, And we ask them to

Teach us, and show us the Way.

We call upon the creatures of the fields and forests
and the seas, our brothers and
sisters the wolves and deer, the eagle and dove,
the great whales and the dolphin,
the beautiful Orca and salmon who share our Northwest home,
and we ask them to

Teach us, and show us the Way.

We call upon all those who have lived on this earth, our
ancestors and our friends,
who dreamed the best for future generations and upon
whose lives our lives are built,
and with thanksgiving, we call upon them to

Teach us, and show us the Way.

And lastly, we call upon all that we hold most sacred, the
presence and power of
the Great Spirit of love and truth which flows through all the
Universe, to be with us to

Teach us, and show us the Way.

—CHINOOK BLESSING LITANY[7]

Our ancestors, who knew their sacred identity with all living forms, created the practice of Hatha yoga. They invented poses that took the forms of different animals and plants to help us joyfully awaken to our participation in the essential life that animates all things. One of the effects of yoga, practiced with this consciousness, is that it frees us from the separateness and loneliness of being only human. It reveals that in the core of our humanity, a divine energy dances, the same energy that appears in and as all of Creation.

Our survival as a species depends upon this recognition of our interrelationship with Creation, and upon the joy, gratitude, and compassion that this awakening arouses in us. The yoga poses that we have selected are ones that can help us taste the truth of our intimate participation in the web of creation in the great yogic text, the Bhagavad Gita. Krishna, the living Divine, tells us this:

> I am the taste of water.
> I am the light of the Sun and the Moon.
> I am the original fragrance of the Earth.
> I am the heat in fire.
> I am the life of all that lives.
> Of lights I am the radiant Sun.
> Among stars I am the Moon.
> Of bodies of water I am the ocean.
> Of immovable things I am the Himalayas.
> Of trees I am the banyan-tree.
> Of weapons I am the thunderbolt.
> Among beasts I am the lion.
> Of purifiers I am the wind.
> Of fishes I am the shark.
> Of flowing rivers I am the Ganges.
> Of seasons I am flower-bearing spring.
> Of secret things I am silence.
> Know that all opulent, beautiful and
> Glorious creations spring from but a spark of my splendor.
>
> —From THE BHAGAVAD GITA[8]

Child's Pose
Adho Mukha Virasana
Sit back on your heels, and then slowly release forward into Child's Pose, resting your forehead on your mat or on a blanket. Place your hands, palms up, by your feet. You may place a bolster under your torso and head to support the front of your spine, or rest your chest upon your thighs. Sink

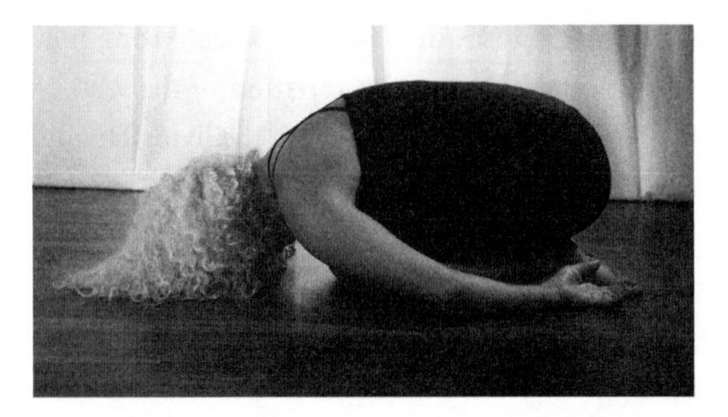

your hips and shoulders down toward the earth, allowing your back to round evenly. Let your forehead relax, letting your thoughts pour like water onto the earth. The skin of your face drops from the bones, and your eyes, jaw, and tongue soften and release.

In the humility, reverence, and surrender of Child's Pose, we open ourselves completely to all of creation. We acknowledge and experience being the embodied child of the Immanent and Transcendent. In this natural human position of prayer, we can find within us the love that radiates from the depths of our heart toward all creatures everywhere. As it is written in the great ancient yogic text, the Mundaka Upanishad,

> The Lord of Love shines in the heart of all,
> Seeing him in all creatures, the wise
> Forget themselves in the service of all.
> The Word is their joy, the Lord is their rest;
> Such as they are the lovers of the Lord.[9]

Arrive in the heart of the present moment. Stay as still as a deer standing silently in the forest, its ears softly quivering, alert to every sound. Listen everywhere, with open spacious awareness, like the deer.

From this vibrant animal stillness, lengthen your arms out in front of you, like a cat stroking the earth, without letting the movement ruffle your mind. Let your arms grow from your heart, sitting bones, and feet. Press your hands down, connecting with and grounding into the darkness of the earth beneath you.

Continue reaching forward as if you were now gently moving through water. Allow your body to undulate softly like a fish. Swim your arms further out onto your mat, lengthening from your belly to your fingers. Let the warm fluid energy you now feel stream evenly to all your cells, awakening your whole body. Feel your oneness with all sea creatures, from the tiniest squiggly amoeba to the majestic blue whale leaping in joy.

Millions of people are now praying in this position of prayer and devotion. Link the human community to the animal world with a prayer for the protection and liberation of all sentient beings everywhere. Your body is now a temple in which your heart sings a silent song of blessing for all creation. As it sings this song, the child is transformed into a nurturing mother.

> May all beings be happy and at their ease! May they be joyous and live in safety!
> All beings, whether weak or strong—omitting none—in high, middle, or low realms of existence, small or great, visible or invisible, near or far away, born or to be born—may all beings be happy and at their ease!
> Even as a mother watches over and protects her child, her only child, so with a boundless mind should one cherish all living beings, radiating friendliness over the entire world, above, below, and all around without limit. So let everyone cultivate a boundless good will toward the entire world, uncramped, free from ill will or enmity.
>
> —The Buddha, from the *MAJJHIMA NIKAYA*[10]

Invoke this spirit of unity with creation to inspire your body-mind throughout the Joy of Creation practice. The following poses will continue to awaken you to your identity with the animal and plant worlds.

Cat/Cow Pose

Slowly come to your hands and knees, balancing on all fours. Lifting your tailbone and head, release your spine down into your body, slowly coming into a slight backbend, the Cow Pose.

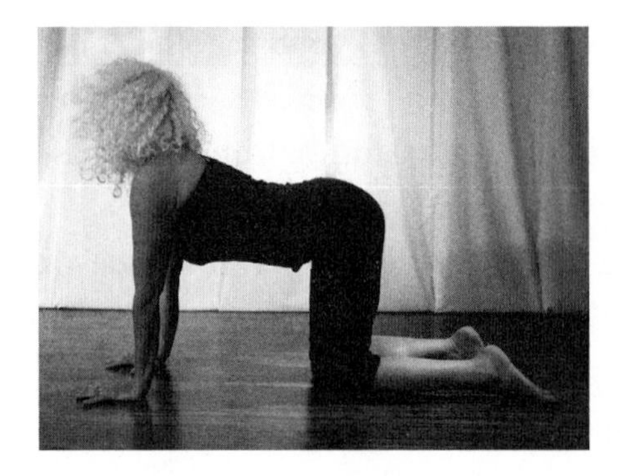
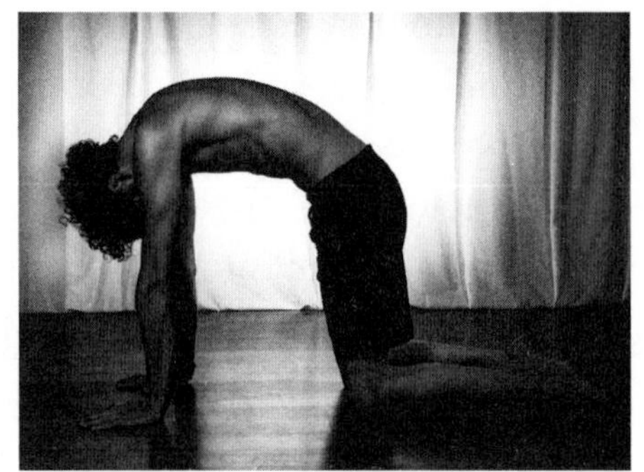

Now draw your spine up into your body, dropping your tailbone and head, and slightly arching your back up into the Cat Pose. Slowly and mindfully move back and forth between Cat and Cow poses, creating an even roundedness of the spine in both shapes, and entering fully into the nature of both animals. Unveil your connection with all the animals that walk this Earth, which Native people recognize as their relations, the four-legged ones.

Trust the wisdom of your body to move as it wants to move. The cat knows exactly when to pounce and when to wait. The cow moves at its own mellow pace. Feel the fluidity of your body, especially the watery belly. Sense how your body, like all bodies, is composed mostly of water and can flow easily from shape to shape.

Downward-facing Dog Pose
Adho Mukha Svanasana
From the hands and knees position, curl your toes under and let your tailbone float up, exploring Downward-facing Dog Pose (for details, see previous instructions on page 69). Let it be a moving, flowing Dog Pose, paws stepping from side to side, tail wagging. Swivel and spiral and enjoy the playfulness of being a dog.

Step one foot forward between your hands to come into a lunge position, and then bring up your other foot between the hands. Coming into the Standing Forward Bend, bend your knees and let your head drop. Your back releases as if rain were pouring down it, moistening and opening your skin.

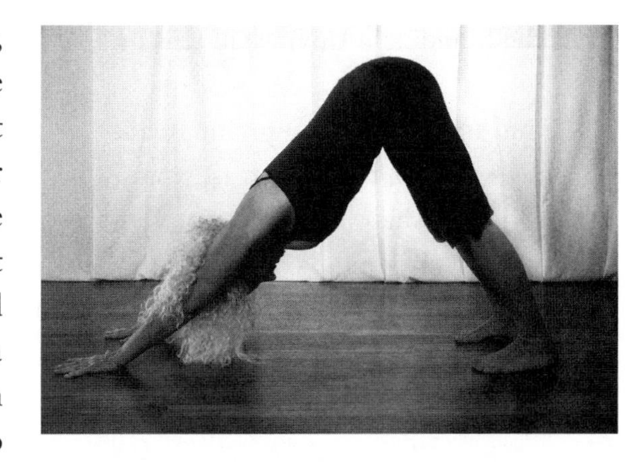

Lift through your belly, and beginning at the base of the spine gradually float up to standing, raising your arms over your head to the sky. Keep your eyes soft and your arms open and embracing. Release into a slight back bend, and then take your hands back to your heart, tenderly pressing the roots of your thumbs into your heart center. Bow your head slightly, dropping your mind into the bed of your heart and softening your eyes in devotion.

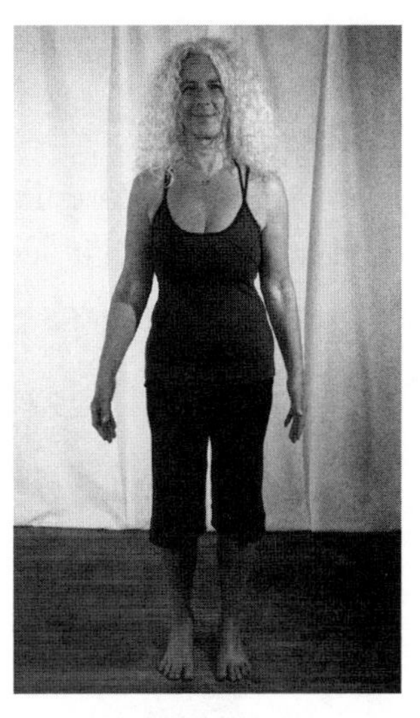

Mountain Pose
Tadasana

Come to Mountain Pose, *Tadasana* (for details, see previous instructions on page 39). Feel your feet firmly on the earth, sensing the strength and lightness in the center of your body. Your legs are earthy and steady; your belly fluid and watery; your heart warm and glowing; and your head empty and spacious. Earth, water, fire, and air unite within your divine human body.

Chanting Om

Remaining in Mountain Pose, the hands joined in prayer position at the heart, now chant the syllable that the yogic sages recognized as the universal sound: the vibration of divine consciousness in all creation. The ancient yogis believed that this holy syllable sprang directly from the Creator's mouth at the beginning of time, infusing all creation with this divine vibratory essence.

As the Mandukya Upanishad tells us,

> Aum stands for the supreme Reality.
> It is a symbol for what was, what is,
> And what shall be. AUM represents also
> What lies beyond past, present, and future.
> Those who know AUM as the Self become the Self;
> Truly they become the Self.
> OM Shanti Shanti Shanti[11]

On an exhalation, let the AUM sound flow and resound throughout your body. Imagine every cell of your body chanting it, and every cell of every living thing echoing and vibrating with your chant.

Tree Pose

Vrksasana

From Mountain Pose slowly shift your weight to your right leg, and steadily send roots through it deep into the ground. Stabilize your right leg, imagining it becoming a tree trunk, and then press the sole of your left foot into the inside of your right thigh. Bring your hands to your heart in the prayer position.

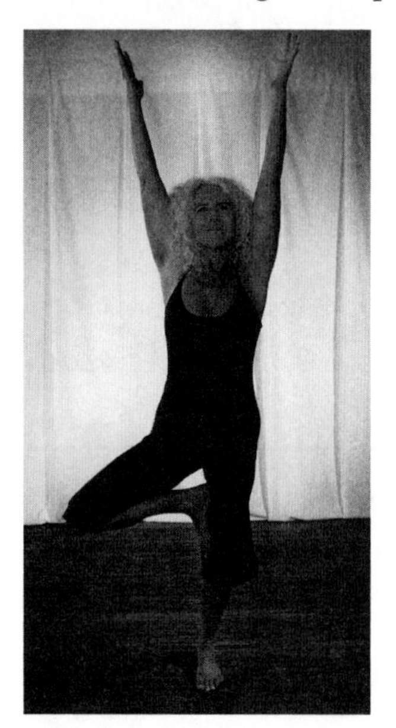

Lift up your belly, as naturally as the sap rises in the spring. Invite that sweet, warm energy to flow into your heart and let your heart open just like a tree breaking into blossom. Lift your arms like branches, your fingers spreading out like leaves opening to the sky. The branches of your arms lift toward the light, while the roots of your legs sink deeply into the earth. Your body in the form of the tree becomes a vibrating channel between earth and sky. Draw your hands together back to your heart, and slowly release your left foot to the floor. Returning to Mountain Pose, drop your tailbone slightly like an anchor before repeating Tree Pose on the other side.

Notice how your body, like a tree, grows upwards toward the light, while spiraling its roots down into the rich dark support of the earth. Return to Mountain Pose whenever you are ready.

Through your identification with the tree that Tree Pose has inspired, enter into the spirit of adoration and renewal that the following Navajo prayer invokes:

> Dark young pine, at the center of the earth originating,
> I have made your sacrifice.
> Whiteshell, turquoise, abalone beautiful,
> Jet beautiful, fool's gold beautiful, blue pollen beautiful,
> Reed pollen, pollen beautiful, your sacrifice I have made.
> This day your child I have become, I say.
>
> Watch over me.
> Hold your hand before me in protection.
> Stand guard for me, speak in defense of me.
> As I speak for you, speak for me.
> May it be beautiful before me.
> May it be beautiful behind me.
> May it be beautiful below me.
> May it be beautiful above me,
> May it be beautiful all around me.
>
> I am restored in beauty
> I am restored in beauty.
> I am restored in beauty.
> I am restored in beauty.[12]

Triangle Pose
Trikonasana

In Triangle Pose you will experience the trinity of body, consciousness, and spirit that you share with all sentient beings, and celebrate your body as a bridge between transcendence and immanence.

Remaining connected to the stability of Mountain Pose, widen your feet about four feet apart. From the earthiness of your feet and legs, spread your arms, lifting them to shoulder height. Turn your left foot in at a 45-degree angle, and your right foot out 90 degrees. To protect your right knee make sure that it turns outward toward the little toe of your right foot.

Inhale, and elongate from the sides of your waist, lengthening your spine to the right as your hips shift to the left, and place your right hand on your right leg or a wooden block. Bring your left hand to your sacrum and let your pelvis rock to and fro a little. You can bend your knees slightly to help you feel the movement of the pelvis. Drawing your sacrum into the body, slowly straighten your legs while moving the tops of your thighbones back behind you.

Feel the energy flowing up through the pelvic floor between your pubic bone and the tailbone. Let it spread up from the belly into the flowering of the heart. Your left arm can now rise up to offer your radiant heart energy to the sky. Both arms are evenly active, equally connecting you to earth and to sky.

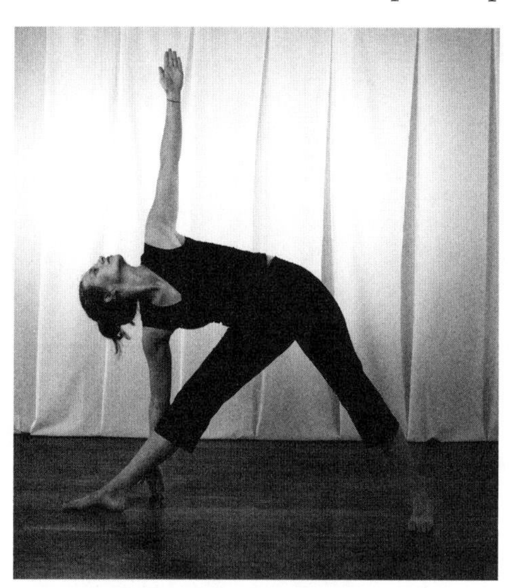

Keeping your legs strong, come up and repeat Triangle Pose to the left side. From the earthiness of the legs, explore the watery nature of the pelvis. It is from the foundation of your legs beneath you that your pelvis is able to release. That freedom moves up into the fire of your heart, and into the empty spaciousness of your head. When you're ready, return to Mountain Pose.

Standing Forward Bend
Uttanasana
From Mountain Pose, bring your hands to the tops of your thighbones and gently slide them back behind you, aligning your hips, knees, and ankles. Lifting your sitting bones, tip your pelvis forward over the tops of your thighs and let your spine evenly round forward into a crescent moon shape. You may bend your knees slightly to protect your back.

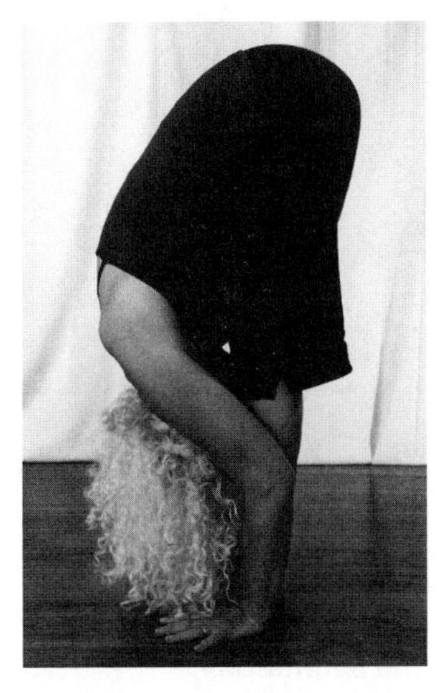

Make a cradle of your arms, and rest your hands on the opposite elbows, or rest your hands on a block, on your legs, or on the floor. Release your head, softening your neck. Relax for a few breaths, surrendering into this pose.

On an exhalation, press down through your feet and up through your belly, rolling up to standing. Your head floats up last, receiving the energy flowing from your feet through your pelvis. You are back to Mountain Pose.

Eagle Pose
Garudasana
From Mountain Pose shift your weight to your left leg, and bend the legs slightly. Lift your right leg, placing your right thigh over your left thigh, and draw your right shin behind your left calf. If it's difficult to balance, you can keep the toes of your right foot on the ground for a while, eventually drawing them around your left calf.

Extend your arms in front of you at shoulder height, palms up. Bend your arms, and draw your left elbow across the right one, pressing the elbows against each other. Try to place the fingers of your right hand in the palm of

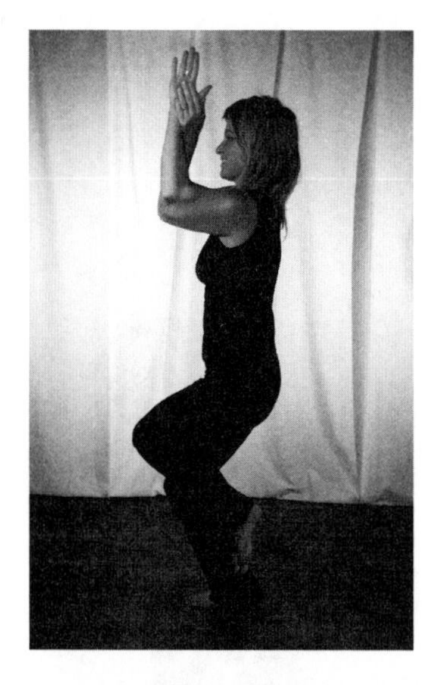

your left hand. Lift your elbows up to eye level, moving your hands away from your head. Scoop through your belly into your heart. Enjoy the expansive release of the wings of your shoulder blades.

Stay three to five breaths then return to Mountain Pose, before repeating Eagle Pose to the other side.

This pose helps you to experience the majesty, concentration, and vitality of the eagle. When you practice, keep your eyes soft, so that you're not coming from the determination of your mind and will. Instead, expand your vision to the spacious perspective of the eagle. Become the eagle, soaring above the world, scanning all of creation with its keen vision and one-pointed concentration.

Sun Salutations

Surya Namaskar

You may wish to add several cycles of the Sun Salutation, to celebrate the light radiating throughout all of creation. Please see the yoga practice for the Joy of Transcendence (page 71) for detailed instructions.

Squatting Pose

Malasana

From Mountain Pose, release your sitting bones down toward the earth, coming into a squatting position. You may place a foam block under your heels for balance.

Many people squat on the earth all day in this position, because they feel grounded and at ease here. Notice how wide open the floor of the pelvis becomes, the first chakra opening to receive energy from the earth.

Sphinx Pose
***Bhujangasana* Modification**

From squatting, slide forward onto your belly, releasing your front body onto the earth. Lengthen your arms out in front of you, like a lion stretching in the desert sun.

In Sphinx Pose, you are invited to savor and claim the full power of the sphinx, tasting the wonder of your own deepest secrets. Let the pose of the sphinx speak to you as it spoke to the Pharaohs, Oedipus, and to Alexander the Great, revealing the magical depth of your identity with all creation.

The ancient Egyptian sphinx is a mythical creature with the face of a human and the body of a lion. This archetypal symbol expresses the serenity and wisdom that are attained when the human being unveils and enters into her identity with all creation. The majesty and mystery of the sphinx have haunted the world's imagination.

Keeping your belly soft, lift your shoulders away from the floor, curling your spine up slightly and sliding your elbows underneath your shoulders. Pressing the palms of your hands down into the earth, widen and lift your collarbones. Roll from leg to leg, drawing your inner legs toward each other until they begin to feel like one leg, grounded in the earth. Slowly and majestically lift your head, smiling serenely. Lift your belly softly toward your heart.

You will feel the warm energy flowing from your lion heart into your head and flooding your human consciousness. Like the sphinx, radiate the lion's compassion and courage to all creatures. Human and animal spiral into each other along the gentle, curling current of the spine.

Slowly release down to the floor, unraveling the cells of your back body. Feel them glow with the serene energy of the heart's nectar. When you are ready, slowly rise up again, repeating Sphinx Pose a few times.

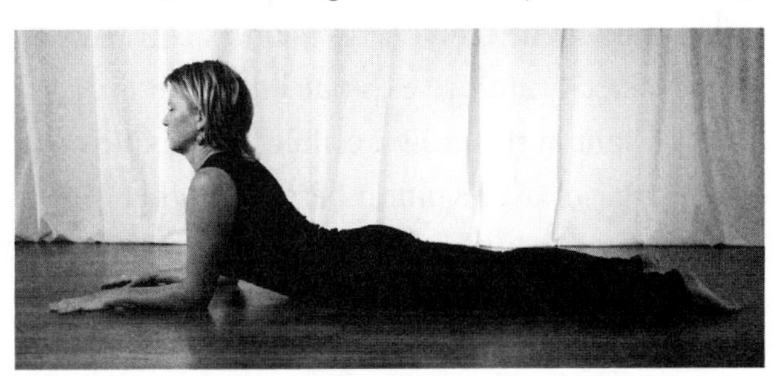

Let the realization of your human/animal identity with all creation awaken your heart center to the sphinx's secret, which Kabir describes with such reverence:

> Near your breastbone there is an open flower
> Drink the honey that is all around that flower.
> Waves are coming in:
> There is so much magnificence near the ocean!
> Listen: Sound of big seashells! Sound of bells!
> Kabir says: Friend, listen, this is what I have to say:
> The guest I love is inside me!
>
> —KABIR[13]

Cobra Pose

Bhujangasana

Soften your belly onto the earth like a golden king cobra. Elongate your spine, and feel it undulating and spiraling throughout its length. Rest here and release your body, with the king cobra's regal confidence, into the dark, rich warmth of the earth below.

In Cobra Pose, you will experience and incarnate the ancient power and sacred wisdom that has in many cultures been associated with the snake. A creature at ease both in the dark worlds of the earth and in the worlds of light, the snake effortlessly fuses the energy and knowledge of both.

In the classical yoga system, the divine energy referred to as "kundalini" is said to be resting dormant at the base of the spine and is depicted as a coiled snake. When this energy is uncoiled, it shoots its fiery power up through all the sacred centers to explode into what is described as a thousand-petaled lotus of light in the crown center. This explosion could be conceived as the divine orgasm of the union between father and mother, transcendence and immanence, and it births the yogi into the bliss energy and knowledge of divine consciousness.

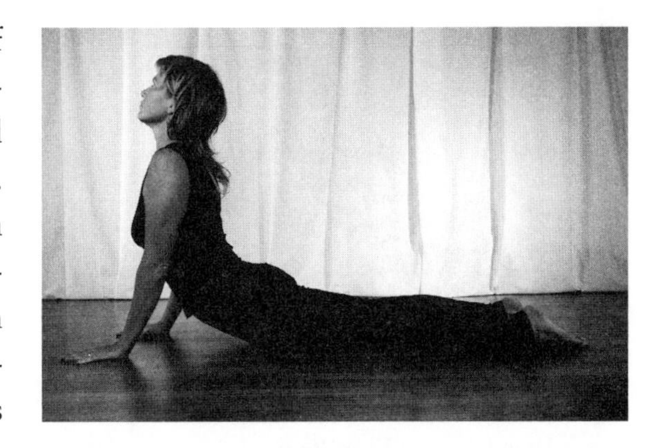

In Hinduism, the god of yogis, Shiva, is often represented with a cobra curled around his right upper arm. This symbolizes the union of spacious sky consciousness with primordial earth energy into which the practice of yoga initiates its devotees.

Slide your hands under your shoulders, and press them down into the earth. Experience the strength of your legs that flows into your pelvis from the arches of your feet. Allow the front of your hips and legs to lengthen, rolling your legs slightly inward. Invite your tailbone toward your pubic bone.

Gently begin to curl your spine by lifting your belly toward the back of your heart, and let your shoulder blades begin to move forward, widening your collarbones. Lift your chest, your spine evenly coiling, without feeling any strain in your low back. Feel the strength of your arms and legs, and the sensuous power of the cobra. From the movement of your royal cobra heart, slowly lift your head. After a few breaths, slowly roll down, softening your belly back to earth. Rest for a few breaths, then elongate and release your spine in Dog Pose. Repeat Cobra Pose a few times.

Feel the snake's smoothness of sensation spreading evenly through your body. In Sanskrit, this evenness of sensation is referred to as *sama,* the root word of "Samadhi." Samadhi is the highest expression of this sameness as absolute consciousness, a consciousness that experiences the One Taste of everything.

Let Cobra Pose consciously awaken you to your own inmost knowledge of the marriage of all opposites, masculine and feminine, earth and sky, human and divine, dark and light, body and spirit, and to the ever-flowing kundalini power that streams from this marriage when it is realized.

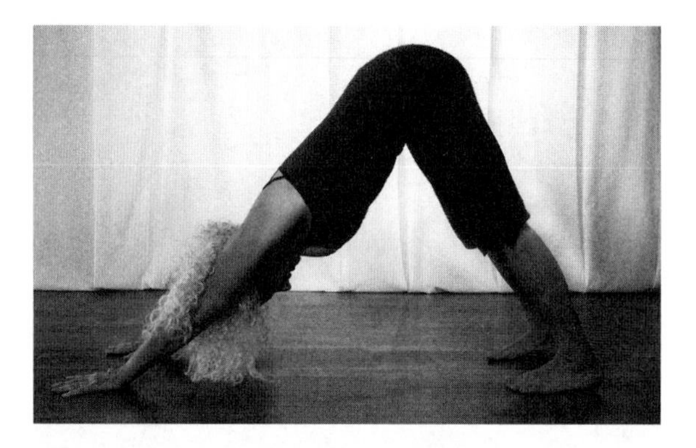

Downward-facing Dog Pose
Adho Mukha Svanasana
From the hands and knees position, curl your toes under and let your tailbone float up, exploring Downward-facing Dog Pose to release the spine after Cobra Pose (for details, see previous instructions on page 106).

Cross-Legged Sitting
Sukhasana
Sit in a simple cross-legged position (refer to page 49 for more details). Elevate your sitting bones on a firm cushion or folded blanket(s), so that your hips are higher than your knees, and your thighbones can drop down from your pelvis. Balance evenly between your sitting bones, your tailbone, and your pubic bone, mapping those four bones like geographical landmarks within the world of your body. Notice how as your lower body descends toward the earth, a warm rebounding rises up through the core channel of your body.

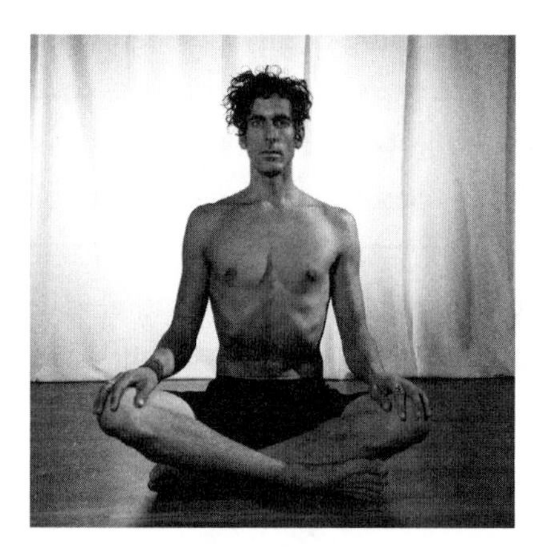

With each exhalation, your pelvic floor domes up into your body like a parachute, and your belly scoops up toward the back of your diaphragm, which also rises with the exhalation. Your heart energy expands while your mind quiets. Notice the subtle dialog between the floor of your pelvis and the crown of your head.

In Cross-legged Sitting Pose consciously remember and integrate, with wonder and gratitude, all the different poses in this yoga practice for celebrating creation, uniting and fusing them within the core of your heart. An ancient Celtic hymn expresses this unity in diversity:

> I am the wind that breathes upon the sea,
> I am the wave on the ocean,
> I am the murmur of leaves rustling,
> I am the rays of the sun,
> I am the beam of the moon and stars,
> I am the power of trees growing
> I am the bud breaking into blossom,
> I am the movement of the salmon swimming,
> I am the courage of the wild boar fighting,
> I am the speed of the stag running,
> I am the strength of the ox pulling the plough,
> I am the size of the mighty oak tree,
> And I am the thoughts of all people
> Who praise my beauty and grace.[14]

Corpse Pose

***Savasana* for Creation**

Lie back onto the sacred earth, your great mother and teacher, with your knees bent and your feet flat on the floor. One at a time, slide your heels out along your mat, surrendering your legs fully back into the earth. Let your breath flow down your legs, moving out through your feet. Sweep your consciousness like a broom from thighs to toes, releasing any holding that you may encounter. Soften your arms out to the sides, palms up. Drop back, releasing your front body into the embrace of your back body; the back body opens into the cauldron of the earth beneath you. As you send roots down

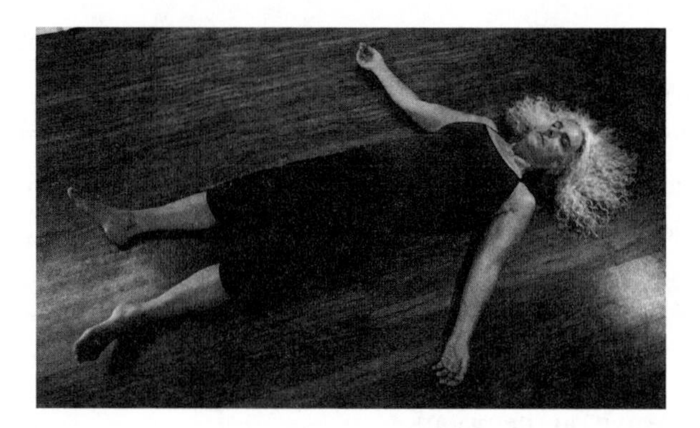

from your own body into the earth, they intermingle and intertwine in the dark mystery of the earth with the roots of all creation.

In this *Savasana,* we merge into the Creation, and the creation teaches us and fills us with its blessings.

Earth teach me stillness
As the grasses are stilled with light.
Earth teach me suffering
As old stones suffer with memory.
Earth teach me humility
As blossoms are humble with beginning.
Earth teach me caring
As the mother who secures her young.
Earth teach me courage
As the tree which stands alone.
Earth teach me limitation
As the ant which crawls on the ground.
Earth teach me freedom
As the eagle which soars in the sky.
Earth teach me resignation
As the leaves which die in the autumn.
Earth teach me regeneration
As the seed which rises in the spring.

Earth teach me to forget myself
As melted snow forgets its life.
Earth teach me to remember kindness
As dry fields weep in the rain.
—UTE PRAYER[15]

Receive all you can learn from the earth as her energy rises up through your body.

Watch your breath with steadiness and ease. The inhalation is absorbed evenly throughout the body, soaking in like moist earth receives a spring rain. Each inhalation flows right through you into the earth. Your exhalation smoothly floats out like dawn mist rises from a lake. Feel your breath joining with the breath of all beings, dissolving together into the spacious sky above you. Feel this peace spreading through your body, and rest here as long as you wish.

Peace be to earth and to airy spaces!
Peace be to heaven, peace to the waters,
Peace to the plants and peace to the trees!
May all the Gods grant me peace!
By this invocation of peace may peace be diffused!
—ATHARVA VEDA 19.9[16]

From the Oneness with all creation that this *Savasana* unveils in you, gently bring your awareness back to your breath, and to the peace and ease flowing through your body. Enjoy the sweet simplicity of resting on the earth, as one divine/human creature among billions of others in creation. Listen to the sounds of creation, near and far, all around you.

Gradually bring yourself fully back from *Savasana,* keeping your belly soft, your breath smooth and easy, your heart open and vulnerable, and your eyes and mind quiet. When you feel ready to move, very slowly roll onto your right side, resting for a few more breaths like a child on its mother's body. Savor the wonder of being created, and so given the grace of embodying the Light.

Slowly come up to a sitting position, and draw your hands to your heart in the Namaste position. Offer your practice to the awakening of all human beings to the divinity of Creation. May we do everything in our power to honor, cherish, and protect all of Creation.

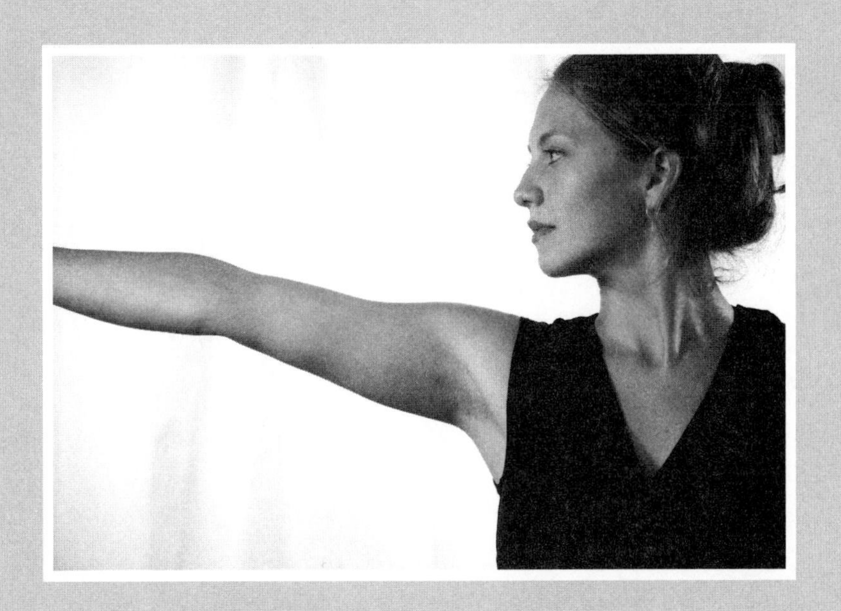

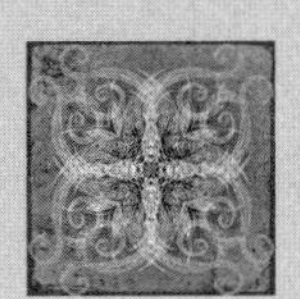 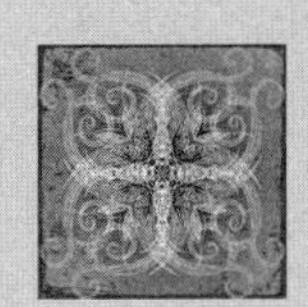 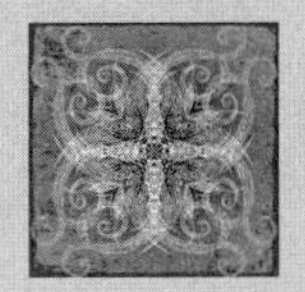

SIX

The Joy of Love for All Beings

The Dalai Lama said to Andrew Harvey, when he interviewed him on the day His Holiness won the Nobel Prize, "The world can only be saved now by everyone trying as hard as possible to love all beings." His Holiness paused and smiled. "This may seem impossible," he said, and then clapped his hands softly. "But with spiritual practice all things are possible. Your Buddha nature is as good as the Buddha's Buddha nature, and who was not embraced by the Buddha's compassion?" And then he quoted from Shantideva's *Mind of the Bodhisattva:* "Those who are unhappy are unhappy because they look out only for themselves. Those who are happy are happy because they seek the joy of others." He paused a long time and then said, "The secret of life is to try to make others happy. People often ask me what is my religion. My religion is kindness."

His Holiness then told a story of how as a young boy he had shot a bird and watched it die, writhing in agony. This had caused him intense pain and regret, he said, and from that moment on, he had felt a special compassion for all animals. Andrew asked him if his religion of kindness embraced even cockroaches and bedbugs. The Dalai Lama looked startled at first and then laughed. "Of course, of course, all creatures, all creatures, even mosquitoes."

A few months later Andrew was teaching in France by the sea. After lecturing all day he was walking on the seashore and saw a tiny bug on a rock, threatened by the incoming tide. The image of the Dalai Lama flooded his mind suddenly, and he picked up the bug and rescued it. He looked at the bug in his palm, and the bug started to dance in an ecstasy of gratitude. Tiny electrical currents shot through his palm from the bug's joy, and for the first time in his life he knew the truth of how love unites all beings in creation.

Yoga Practice Sequence to Celebrate the Joy of Love for All Beings

- Sun Salutations – *Surya Namaskar*
- Supported Heart Opener
- Back Release

- Sphinx Pose – *Bhujangasana* modification
- Cobra Pose – *Bhujangasana*
- Hero Pose – *Virasana*
- Camel Pose – *Ustrasana*
- Pelvis Rocks
- Bridge Pose – *Setu Bandhasana*
- Upward-facing Bow Pose – *Urdhva Dhanurasana*
- Bridge Pose – *Setu Bandhasana*
- Reclined Leg Release – *Supta Padanguthasana*
- Reclined Back Twist – *Jathara Parivartanasana*
- Back Releases
- Legs Up Wall Pose – *Viparita Karani*
- *Savasana*

Although yoga may seem like a solitary practice, this inner journey can birth a love for one's own being that leads gracefully to an all-embracing love for all beings. Patanjali taught how important it is for the yogi to cultivate the qualities of the heart: "friendliness, compassion, gladness, and joy" (Yoga Sutras, I-33).[1] B. K. S. Iyengar believes that "without these, we have not achieved the true yoga of Patanjali."[2] Iyengar explains further, "You have to create love and affection for your body, for what it can do for you. Love must be incarnated in the smallest pore of the skin, the smallest cell of the body, to make them intelligent, so they can collaborate with all the other ones in the big republic of the body. This love must radiate from you to others."[3] Someone who is healing and growing in self-love naturally begins to feel unconditional love for all beings. As Walt Whitman wrote in one of the fragments that precedes *Leaves of Grass,* "I celebrate myself to celebrate you, I say the same word for every man and woman alive, And I say that the soul is not greater than the body, And I say that the body is not greater than the soul."[4]

Patanjali makes clear that when this sacred intelligence of the cells is awakened, and the collaboration Iyengar describes is deepened and extended, the yogi begins to love the republic of his own body and to care for all beings in the vast republic of the world. The cells of one's own body awaken to both vibrant physical health and to the vibrant spiritual health of compassion, resonating in loving union with the cells of all bodies in a dynamic dance of love-energy.

Yoga takes both the emotional and the spiritual experience of love down into the deepest recesses of the body, and marries it with each cell, illumining the entire being. Then love reveals itself, not as a duty, not as a rare achievement, not as emotion only, nor even as the highest form of spiritual knowledge, but as the essential glowing energy of all life.

As the Shvetashvatara Upanishad proclaims:

> The Self is hidden in the hearts of all,
> As butter lies hidden in cream. Realize
> The Self in the depths of meditation—
> The Lord of Love, supreme Reality,
> Who is the goal of all knowledge.
> This is the highest mystical teaching;
> This is the highest mystical teaching.[5]

The Upanishads describe this realization as the highest mystical teaching, because when it is unshakeable all duality evaporates, leaving only knowledge, existence, and bliss *(Sat/Chit/Ananda)*.

Awakening to the presence of the Self in every cell of your own body as described by the Upanishads awakens you to the presence of the Self in all bodies, and to the love that the Self radiates naturally to and from all the forms of its own manifestation. This awakening usually begins in the opening of the heart center and then illumines the spiritual intellect. When, through conscious yoga practice, it starts to permeate and saturate, as Iyengar says, "the smallest pore of the skin, the smallest cell of the body,"[6] it immeasurably grounds, deepens, and expands the power of the realization.

Compassion flows naturally when this awareness is established. This Self-realization manifests itself, the yogic sages make clear, in an ever-deepening spontaneous desire to serve all beings in love, as the following Buddhist prayer expresses.

> Let us live joyfully.
> Let us form a community of love, in a world full of hatred.
> Let us live without any kind of hatred.
> Let us live joyfully.
> Let us form a community of spiritual health, in a world full of illness.
> Let us live without any kind of spiritual disease.
> Let us live joyfully.
> Let us form a community of peace, in a world full of rivalry.
> Let us live without any kind of rivalry.
> Let us live joyfully.
> Let us form a community which possesses nothing.
> Let us live on spiritual bliss, radiating spiritual light.
>
> —From the *DHAMMAPADA*[7]

Sun Salutations

Surya Namaskar

This sequence of asanas celebrating the joy of love for all beings is designed to deepen your experience of the presence of the Self within your body, and to help you extend the Self's compassion to all beings. It invites the sun of your heart to shine with awakened love, tenderness, and gratitude.

Begin with a few Sun Salutations (See page 71) to awaken the radiance of the heart center. Practice with reverent devotion, offering your heart in tender love to all beings. This practice is an opportunity to hear the whispering of your heart.

Come down to a squatting position, bringing your hands together in prayer position in front of the heart. After a few breaths here, slowly release your sitting bones to the floor, and lengthen your legs out in front of you. Place your elbows on the floor, and elongate your spine back down toward the earth, resting back onto your mat.

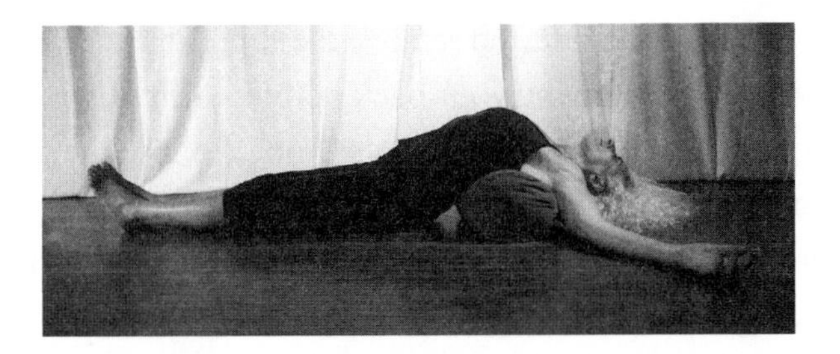

Supported Heart Opener

Lying back with your knees bent and resting on each other, place the soles of your feet flat on the floor, parallel to each other. Put a low foam block, a folded blanket, or a rolled-up yoga mat under your shoulder blades, to elevate them and release your heart center. Lengthen your arms out to the sides, feeling your heart energy flow through your upturned palms.

Release your back down into the earth, and do a few gentle pelvic rocks. Feel your sacrum, the sacred bone, and align it with the same attention that a jeweler would give to carefully placing a diamond into an exquisite setting.

Feel your breath flowing into the space around your heart. Relax and listen to the voice of your heart. Notice, with honesty and clarity, what you are feeling right now, with a willingness to see the shadows as well as the light. Softening your eyes with each inhalation, keep letting your breath drift down toward your heart. Inhale, softening your eyes. Exhale, and rest back into your heart. If you feel any tenderness or pain around your heart, gently open to it and gradually explore it.

> Don't surrender your loneliness so quickly.
> Let it ferment and season you as few human or divine
> ingredients can.
> Something missing in my heart tonight has made my eyes so soft,
> my voice so tender,
> my need of God absolutely clear.
>
> —HAFIZ[8]

Now slowly roll to the side and remove the support underneath you, lying back on the floor and allowing your back body to melt down into the earth. Keep your knees bent and feet flat on the floor. Follow the thread of your breath down into the back of your heart, the space between your shoulder blades, where pain or grief is often stored. Relax and breathe into this opening place underneath your heart.

The Sufis say that spiritual awakening may be experienced like a kiss on the back of the heart. This is a place no human can touch, and where the Beloved expresses its intimate compassion for you. This is the kiss you have been waiting for all your life, the kiss of the Beloved, in the mysterious depth of your own body.

As you open to the Divine, you will increasingly feel the bliss of this tender kiss within you, which your breath spreads like a soft fire through your heart to all the cells of your body. This fire may feel at times almost painful, like a longing or burning. Stay with whatever arises, listening to the deepest message of your heart.

LOVE AFTER LOVE
The time will come
when, with elation,
you will greet yourself arriving
at your own door, in your own mirror,
and each will smile at the other's welcome,

and say, sit here. Eat.
You will love again the stranger who was your self.
Give wine. Give bread. Give back your heart
to itself, to the stranger who has loved you

all your life, whom you ignored
for another, who knows you by heart.
Take down the love letters from the bookshelf,

the photographs, the desperate notes,
peel your own image from the mirror.
Sit. Feast on your life.
—DEREK WALCOTT[9]

Back Release

Now cross your shins and let your knees fall out to the sides. With infinite compassion, place your hands over your heart, as if to cradle it.

Notice whatever veils of fear, pain, loss, disappointment, or grief still shroud your heart. Breathe into your heart and hands, and with each breath see the mist of those veils beginning to evaporate, and the sun of your heart starting to shine through. Listen to your own timeless wisdom speaking to you from your heart.

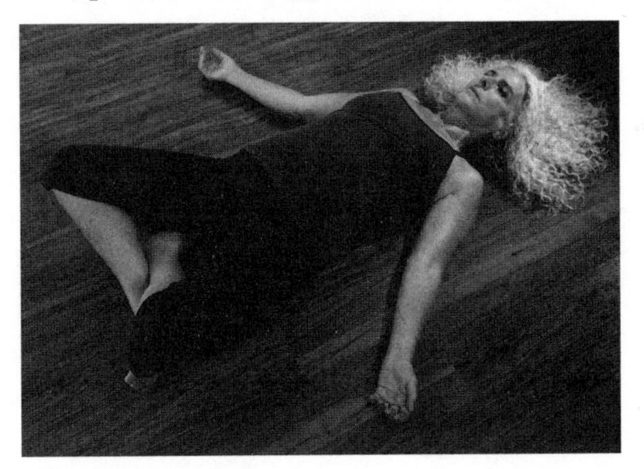

Have patience with everything unresolved in your heart
And try to love the questions themselves . . .
Don't search for the answers,
They could not be given to you now,
Because you would not be able to live them.
And the point is, to live everything.
Live the questions now.
Perhaps then, someday in the future,
You will gradually, without even noticing it,
Live your way into the answer.
—RAINER MARIA RILKE[10]

Now turn to your right side and rest for a few breaths. Then roll over onto your belly, feeling it soften onto Mother Earth, as if you were a young child resting on your mother's body. Notice the natural inclination of your heart and belly to soften and release.

Sphinx Pose
***Bhujangasana* modification**
Releasing your front body onto the earth, lengthen your arms out in front of you, like a lion stretching in the desert sun.

In Sphinx Pose, you are invited to savor and claim the full power of the sphinx, tasting the wonder and mystery of your own deepest secrets. Let the pose of the sphinx speak to you as it spoke to the Pharaohs, Oedipus, and Alexander the Great, revealing the magical depth of your identity with all creation.

The ancient Egyptian sphinx is a mythical creature with the face of a human and the body of a lion. This archetypal symbol expresses the serenity and wisdom that are attained when the human being unveils and enters into her identity with all creation. The majesty and mystery of the sphinx have haunted the world's imagination.

Keeping your belly soft, lift your shoulders away from the floor, curling your spine up slightly and sliding your elbows underneath your shoulders. Pressing the palms of your hands down into the earth, widen and lift your collarbones. Roll from leg to leg, drawing your inner legs toward each other until they begin to feel like one leg, grounded in the earth. Slowly and majestically lift your head, smiling serenely. Lift your belly softly toward your heart.

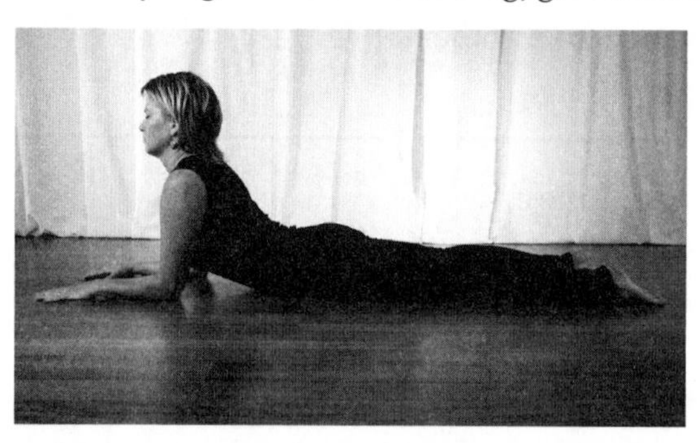

You will feel the warm energy flowing from your lion heart into your head and flooding your human consciousness. Like the sphinx, radiate the lion's compassion and courage to all creatures. Human and animal spiral into each other along the gentle, curling current of the spine.

Slowly release back down to the floor, unraveling the cells of your back body. Feel them glow with the serene energy of the heart's nectar. When you are ready, slowly rise up again, repeating Sphinx Pose a few times, slowly and peacefully.

Let the realization of your human/animal identity with all creation awaken your heart center to the sphinx's secret.

Cobra Pose
Bhujangasana

Soften your belly onto the earth like a golden king cobra. Elongate your spine, and feel it undulating and spiraling throughout its length. Rest here and release your body, with the king cobra's regal confidence, into the dark, rich warmth of the earth below.

In Cobra Pose, you will experience and incarnate the ancient power and sacred wisdom that has in many cultures been associated with the snake. A creature at ease both in the dark worlds of the earth and in the worlds of light, the snake effortlessly fuses the energy and knowledge of both.

In the classical yoga system, the divine energy referred to as "kundalini" is said to be sleeping at the base of the spine; it is depicted as a coiled snake. When this energy is uncoiled, it shoots its fiery power up through all the sacred centers to explode into what is described as a thousand-petaled lotus of light in the crown center. This explosion could be conceived as the divine orgasm of the union between father and mother, transcendence and immanence, and it births the yogi into the bliss energy and knowledge of divine consciousness.

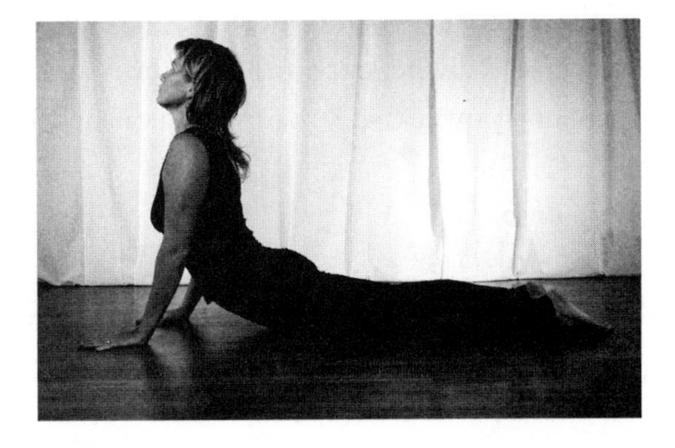

In Hinduism, the god of yogis, Shiva, is often represented with a cobra curled around his right upper arm. This symbolizes the union of spacious sky consciousness with primordial earth energy into which the practice of yoga initiates its devotees.

Slide your hands under your shoulders, and press them down into the earth. Experience the strength of your legs that flows into your pelvis from the arches of your feet. Allow the fronts of your hips and legs to lengthen, rolling your legs slightly inward. Invite your tailbone toward your pubic bone.

Gently begin to coil your spine by lifting your belly toward the back of your heart, and let your shoulder blades begin to move forward, widening your collarbones. Lift your chest, your spine evenly coiling, without feeling any strain in your low back. Feel the strength of your arms and legs, and the sensuous power of the cobra rising. From the movement of your royal cobra heart, slowly lift your head. After a few breaths, gradually roll down, softening your belly back to earth. Rest for a few breaths, then elongate and release your spine in Dog Pose. Repeat Cobra Pose a few more times.

Feel the snake's smoothness of sensation spreading evenly through your body. In Sanskrit, this evenness of sensation is referred to as *sama,* the root word of "Samadhi." Samadhi is the highest expression of this sameness as absolute consciousness, a consciousness that experiences the One Taste of everything.

Let Cobra Pose consciously awaken you to your own inmost knowledge of the marriage of all opposites, masculine and feminine, earth and sky, human and divine, dark and light, body and spirit, and to the ever-flowing kundalini power that streams from this marriage when it is realized.

Hero Pose

Virasana

After Cobra Pose, rise to your hands and knees and then come to Downward-facing Dog Pose for a few breaths, elongating and releasing your spine. Bring your knees to the floor, and sit back on your heels in Hero Pose (See page

78). Lift your arms to the sides, palms facing up. Breathing into your heart center, sweep the arms overhead to join your palms in prayer. Keeping your heart lifted, slowly release your hands down to your heart. Listen to the message from your heart. After a few breaths, rest your hands on your thighs, feeling your legs, sitting bones, and feet melting into the earth.

Camel Pose
Ustrasana

> Him to whom you pray is closer to you than the neck of your camel.
>
> —MUHAMMAD

Sitting back on your heels, press down through your feet and legs. Lift your sitting bones up away from your heels. Anchor your pelvis by dropping your tailbone toward the earth. Curl your toes under and open the arches of your feet. Bring your hands prayerfully to your heart. With your inhalation lift your heart; with your exhalation, curl your tailbone slightly forward and elongate your spine.

Stream energy down into the earth from your hips to your knees. Your belly lifts up toward your heart center, and your collarbones rise and spread wide. Reach your fingertips back and place them on your heels. If that is too far to reach, place your hands on blocks, leave your hands on your heart, or put them on the backs of your legs.

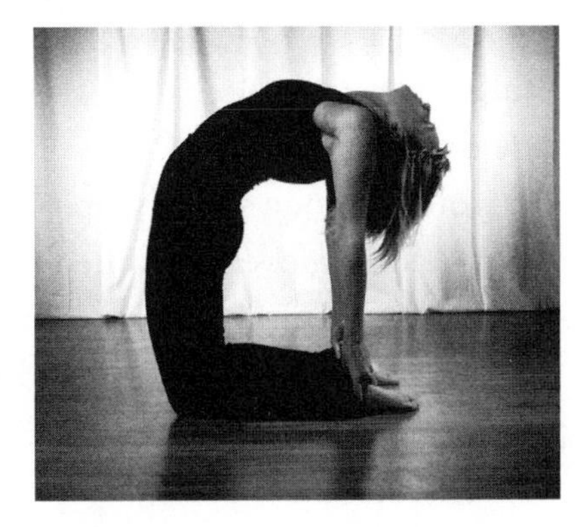

Without compressing your lower back, keep lifting your heart and feel it expanding and spreading in luminous space.

Open the chalice of your heart so that the divine honey can pour in, and drink the honey of your heart. Send the joy of this pose out to all beings as an offering of your love.

> Now may every living thing, young or old,
> Weak or strong, living near or far, known or unknown, living or departed or yet unborn,
> May every living thing be full of bliss.
> —THE BUDDHA[11]

Stay in this heart-releasing position of love and joy for a few breaths, and then slowly return your sitting bones to your heels, drawing your tailbone toward the floor to lengthen your lower back. Keep your heart lifted, radiating the golden light of compassion in all directions. Repeat Camel Pose *(Ustrasana)* several times, returning to Hero Pose *(Vajrasana)* to rest.

Pelvic Rocks

Roll onto your back, bending your knees and placing your feet parallel to each other, hip width apart. Press them down, embedding them into the floor. Notice the earthiness of your feet and the strength of your legs. Feel this Mother Earth energy lovingly infuse the minutest channels of your leg bones, and follow this warm flow up into your pelvis. Gently rock your pelvis back and forth, letting the earth massage your low back.

Bridge Pose

Setu Bandhasana

Lift your tailbone slightly up off the floor, curling it toward your pubic bone. Let this movement initiate the lift of your sitting bones off the floor. A flow of energy, originating from the arches of your feet, enters the sacred space between your tailbone and your pubic bone. This energy lifts your belly and hips up from the floor, your belly floating toward the sky and your heart rising.

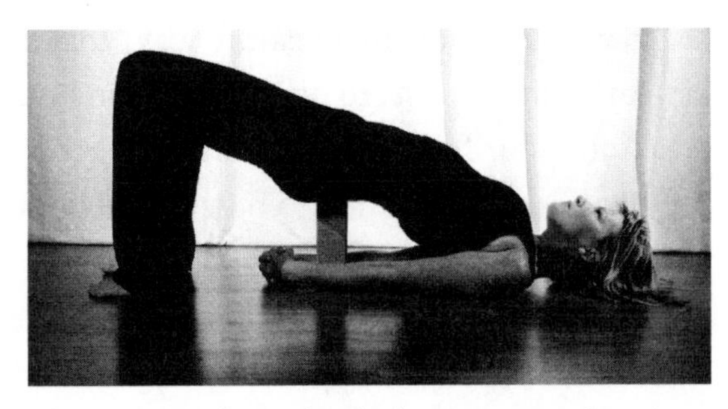

Now gently roll down onto the floor, first coming down between your shoulder blades, then the back of your waist, and then your tailbone, uncurling each vertebra mindfully as if your spine were a precious string of pearls. Notice how your front body begins to soften into the embrace of your broad back body. As the heart energy of the Bridge Pose flows into your arms, press them strongly down into the earth. The strength of your arms and legs supports your spine in a rainbow arc, while your belly and heart float softly on this luminous arc. Allow your spine to relax into a gently rounded crescent moon; then slowly return back to earth and rest. In this pose you experience the body celebrating its inherent nature as a bridge between earth and sky, as a child of the Mother-Father.

Repeat Bridge Pose a few times, letting this heart energy brim over into your head as your mind floods with its tender, loving warmth. (See page 46 for more details on this pose.)

Upward-facing Bow Pose
Urdvha Dhanurasana

(Do not practice this pose with back or wrist injury, during the last six months of pregnancy, or during the menstrual flow.)

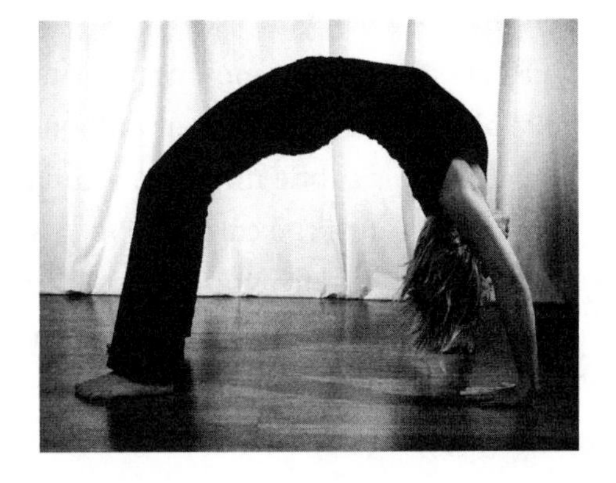

In this ecstatic pose, the absolutely open heart is supported by the strength and calm of the absolutely balanced body. It symbolizes the necessity of a strong, unwavering connection with the earth beneath you as the foundation from which you can whole-heartedly offer yourself to the Beloved.

To give to others in a healthy way, you need to be grounded in yourself. Similarly, in this pose, to offer yourself in love you first sink your roots down deep into your feet and into the earth. From that grounded security, firmly centered in the immanent, you can fully open yourself in love to the transcendent.

The asana is itself the manifestation of the Sacred Marriage. It gives us a sublime and practical key to entering the fullness of the marriage: establish yourself in the depths of your body as you simultaneously open your whole heart, mind, and being to Love. A tree cannot grow into its full majesty unless its roots are entwined deep into the earth.

Doing the pose with this awareness will awaken you to the vibrant balance called for by a life of authentic love. When you open yourself to the infinite wellspring of love energy that is always flowing within you, loving others comes naturally.

Explore this pose as an offering from the core of your heart and body, rather than trying to push into it as a test of your will or endurance. As Iyengar writes, "When you do the asana correctly the Self opens by itself; this is divine yoga."[12]

Experiment carefully with this intense backbend. Lying on your back, bend your knees and place your feet parallel and hip width apart near your sitting bones. Bring your hands underneath your shoulders, fingers pointing back toward your heels and turned a bit to the outside. Your hands can be placed slightly wider than your shoulders, so that your elbows will stay over your hands when you rise up.

Rock your pelvis, moving your tailbone toward your pubic bone; then your pubic bone toward your tailbone. On an exhalation, curl your tailbone up, letting this subtle movement initiate the rising of your hips off the floor. Move down into the earth through your hands and arms, and draw your shoulder blades into your body, lifting your chest. You may wish to first lightly rest the crown of your head on the floor, being careful that you don't compress your neck.

Engage your shoulder blades into the back ribs, and your arm bones firmly into your shoulder sockets. Make sure your feet and legs are parallel and hip width apart. Strongly press down through your hands and feet, and unroll into a full backbend. Stay for a few breaths, then slowly and mindfully release down. Repeat a few more times, practicing rolling your spine up rather than forcing it up into your body.

Move down through your legs, and open the fronts of your hips and thighs. Lift your tailbone up, releasing your sacrum deeply into your body and elongating through your lower back. Allow your spine to curl into an even roundedness, supported by the strength of your arms and legs. Keep your belly soft, your heart lifting, and your breath easy and flowing.

Come down to the floor whenever you feel ready, resting and then repeating the pose a few times. When you release down to earth, rest and radiate out to all sentient beings the intense energy that has flooded you. This energy comes from both the strong support of the earth and from the transcendent shining its light down upon you.

> O love, O pure, deep love, be here, be now, be all.
> Worlds dissolve into your stainless, endless radiance.
> Frail living leaves burn with you brighter than cold stars.
> Make me your servant, your breath, your core.
>
> —RUMI[13]

Bridge Pose

Setu Bandhasana

After Upward-facing Bow Pose, explore another gentle Bridge Pose (See page 46) to release your spine. Experiment with lengthening your fingers toward your heels, turning your palms up, clasping your hands, or placing your hands under your hips. Practice without any pushing or struggle, lifting up with ease and staying only as long as feels right.

When you come back down to the floor after Bridge Pose, practice a few gentle pelvic tilts, releasing and relaxing your back and belly. Allow your belly to stay quiet, like a still pool deep in the middle of the forest. Sense the

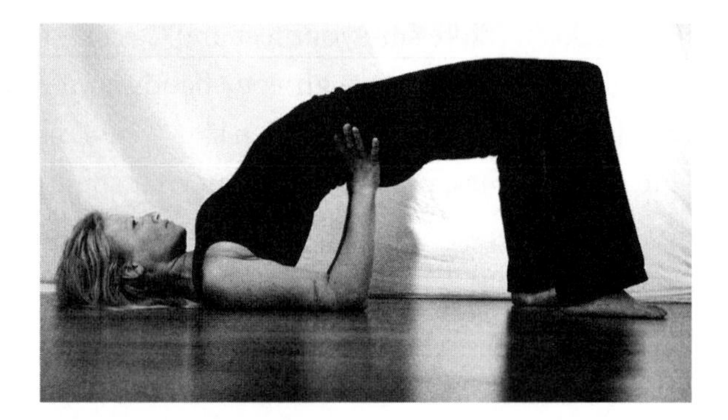

warm glowing fire of your heart. Feel the joy of opening your body so freely, and of opening your heart so naturally to love.

Reclined Leg Release
Supta Padanguthasana
Hug your right knee gently to your chest. Notice how the right side of your back opens and releases, and your internal organs on the right side soften. Slowly lengthen your left leg, moving out through your left heel and awakening your left foot.

Allow energy to spread throughout your entire body into every cell. Hold your right leg, or place a strap around your right foot and slowly straighten that leg, holding the strap with both hands and resting your shoulders on the floor. Stay fully present throughout your whole body in this pose, rather than just concentrating on your leg.

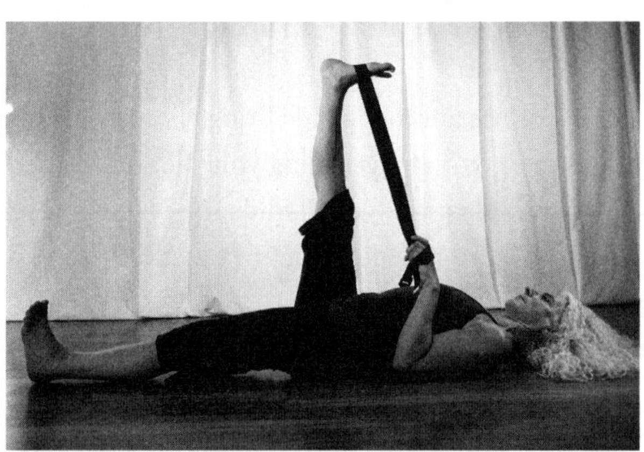

Keep your left leg dropping down toward the floor, elongating through your left heel and releasing your low back. Your left leg rolls slightly to the inside, your right leg a bit to the outside, to maintain an even alignment of your pelvis.

After at least five breaths, fold your right knee back to your chest, and then place the sole of your right foot on the floor. Slowly draw the heel of this foot down your mat, lengthening and releasing your right leg. Rest a few breaths before repeating this pose on the other side.

Reclined Back Twist
Jathara Parivartanasana

Lying on your back, exhale, and draw your right knee up toward your chest. Move slowly and consciously, feeling your back opening and releasing to the earth. Relax the skin on your face and release your lower jaw. With each inhalation, soften your eyes. Lengthen your left leg onto the floor, elongating through your left heel. Strongly awaken your left foot, as if it were standing on the wall across from you. Spread your heart energy all the way down into both feet.

Now slowly roll your right knee across your body toward your left side, resting it on a folded blanket or block. Gently place your left hand on your right knee. Take your right hand back to your lower back. With the exhalation, feel how your tailbone slightly lengthens and delicately moves toward your pubic bone. With your inhalation, the pubic bone moves toward your tailbone. Notice the subtle dancing energy between your pubic bone and your tailbone.

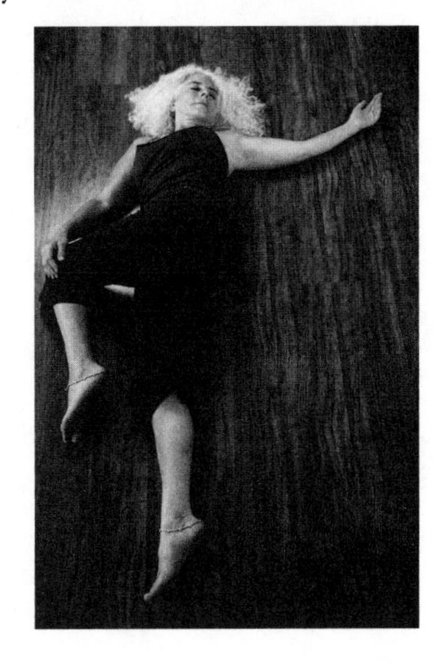

From your pelvic floor, draw your awareness up toward your heart. Inhaling, fill your chest, and exhaling, release your right arm behind you. Notice how the area around your heart feels as you move your arm. Your belly lifts up toward your heart, and your heart energy radiates and streams out your arm.

If you feel any tension or tenderness in your back, modify this position so that it feels easier and more comfortable. You can take your right hand to your back and massage it. Bring a healing touch to wherever your body needs it, and notice how soothing the touch of your hand can be on your own body.

Imagine a golden light entering your open heart. Your heart is like a glowing chalice receiving the divine golden honey pouring into it.

Feel how the inhalation widens the area around your heart, and the exhalation deeply softens your heart space. Draw your body and breath together with the gentle focus of your mind.

In the Reclined Back Twist, your heart blossoms open like a flower of light radiating love energy throughout the channel of your arm and out through your fingertips behind you, into the world. In this heart-releasing and heart-expanding position, imagine that you are receiving a downpouring of compassionate light from the Beloved, like a golden rain upon your body, and radiate it outward to all beings. Pray that this golden love energy, the energy of the sacred heart, can descend as peace on all sentient beings.

When you are ready to move, slowly come back to the center, drawing both knees up to your chest. As your back body widens and releases, rock gently back and forth, resting here a few breaths before exploring the twist to the other side.

In the Reclined Back Twist, the intense and ecstatic offering of the heart in the Camel and Upward-facing Bow poses is experienced at a gentler depth. The passionate and fiery energy of those poses is distilled into a tender experience of love and union with all things. Through this pose, the passionate fire of divine love at its most exposed is alchemized into a quiet and blissful tenderness that is the foundation for a ceaseless flow of love-energy.

St. John of the Cross describes the transformation of the heart in the fire of love as having three stages. First, the log of the ordinary self, covered with the moss and lichens of confusion, is placed in the fire and starts to spit and crackle as it is purified. Then, as the fire of love enters the log more and more completely, it flares up in exuberant flame. Lastly, in the third stage, the flames of passion transform into the embers of an infinitely soft and tender glow that, as St. John says, "helps us enter the tenderness of the life of God."[14]

When it feels like the same amount of time on the second side, slowly return to the center, hugging both knees to your chest.

Once you have experienced, through grace and by your practice of yoga, the realization of this holy and tender absorption into love, you discover that it is from this soft fire that the calm strength and energy flows to radiate love outward to all beings. The paradox revealing itself here is that by reaching the most intimate union within ourselves, we find the source of a deathless power to continue loving others in boundless compassion. As Rumi invites us,

> Each moment from all sides rushes to us the call to love.
> We are running to contemplate its vast green field.
> Do you want to come with us?
> This is not the time to stay at home,
> But to go out and give yourself to the garden.
> The dawn of joy has arisen,
> And this is the moment of union, of vision.
>
> —RUMI[15]

Back Releases

These positions offer many options to explore letting go and resting. Lie on your back and hug your knees toward you. Rock from side to side, or from top to bottom, massaging your back on the floor. Cross your legs as if sitting cross-legged, with one shin on top of the other, releasing your knees toward the floor. Cross your legs with the other shin on top, and bring awareness to your breath.

Visualize your heart flowering open with your inhalation, and your belly releasing and relaxing with your exhalation, each breath gently cradling the

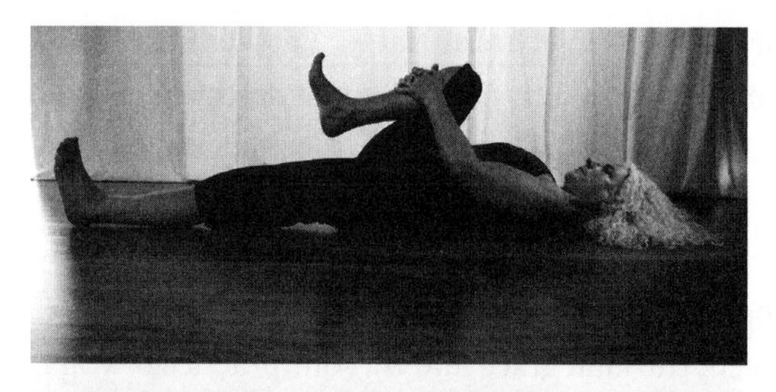

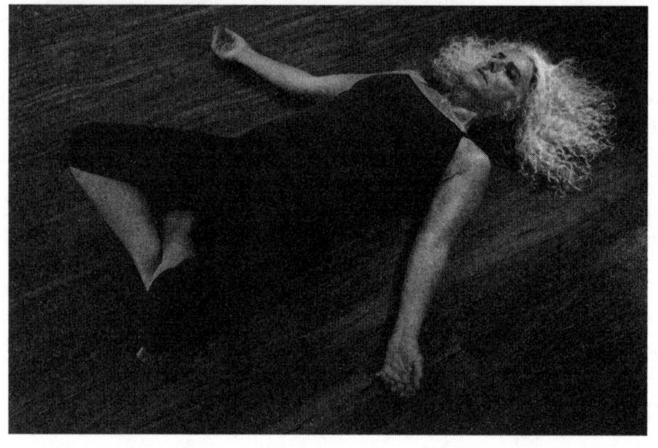

heart. Rest your knees on each other, your feet flat on the floor, or put the soles of your feet together. Allow your back to melt into the earth.

Legs Up Wall Pose
Viparita Karani
Sit with one hip close to a wall, then swing around and put your legs up the wall. Your back can rest on the floor, or you can place a support under your hips and chest to elevate your torso slightly while your shoulders rest on the floor. This creates a gentle roundedness throughout your chest. If it feels like your chin is lifting too much, place a small pillow under your head and neck to support the curve of your neck, and adjust your forehead so that it's higher than your chin.

Spread your arms to the sides, opening your heart center, and turn your palms up. Release the tops of your thighbones toward the wall, softening your belly with each exhalation. If your legs or back feel uncomfortable, adjust the distance of your hips from the wall, or bend your legs slightly. An eye pillow softens the gaze inward.

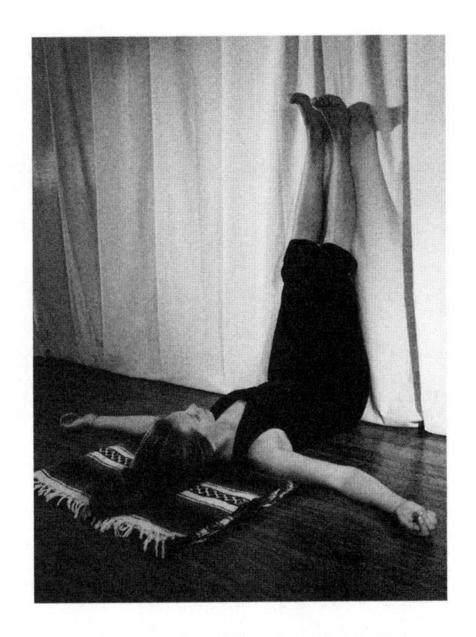

Observe how tension and tiredness drain down your legs, and energy flows like a waterfall into the quiet pool of your pelvis, brimming back into your heart and head. The breath releases your chest, and heart energy flows freely in all directions, permeating your mind. Rest in the joy of release, your heart awake in pure love for all beings. Absorb these holy words from the Upanishads:

> This is the spirit that is in my heart, smaller than a grain of rice, or a grain of barley, or a grain of mustard seed, or a grain of canary-seed, or the kernel of a grain of canary-seed; this is the spirit that is in my heart, greater than the Earth, greater than the sky, greater than heaven itself, greater than all these worlds. This is the spirit that is in my heart.[16]

***Savasana* for Love for All Beings**

Lie back on the floor with your knees up and feet on the floor, and bring your hands under your kidneys, feeling them softening back into your hands. With your hands, draw the skin on your lower back down toward your sitting bones, lengthening your lower back. Spread your back body down onto the floor, letting yourself sink back.

Place an eye pillow over your eyes. Slowly lengthen out your legs, feeling their warmth and heaviness as they release and relax back into the floor. Let them melt back, and consciously move down your legs through your hips, through your thighs, knees, shins, calves, ankles, and feet, sweeping away any holding out the arches of your feet, so that your legs can totally drop back. As your legs soften, your belly releases, and your

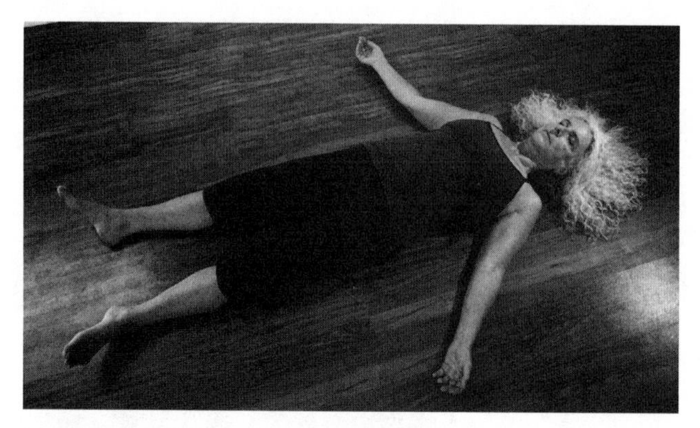

heart sun opens and shines.

Notice how easily and gently your body absorbs your inhalation, like a soft rain falling upon moist earth. Your exhalation floats up, like mist rising. Soften back, sinking into yourself. Let go for now of anything you've been holding, letting thoughts float away like clouds, leaving no trace. Release, now, all illusion of separateness, so that you are able to open into the vast spaciousness of love for all beings. From that spaciousness, pray that the infinite love with which you are becoming one heals and brings peace to all beings.

Let the cells of your body now absorb this prayer:

> Make me
> A still place of light
> A still place of love
> Of you
> Your light radiating
> Your love vibrating
> Your touch and your healing
> Far flung and near
> To the myriads caught
> In darkness, in sickness
> In lostness, in fear
> Make a heart-center here,
> Light of the World.
>
> —PRAYER FROM MALLING ABBEY, DENMARK[17]

With the boundaries of your body dissolved like salt in water, float as the ocean of love, waves of light softly breaking in all directions.

Imagine you are lying on a raft of light, your body glowing, light pouring down from the Beloved like golden rain. From the altar of your raft, your body radiates its own golden light as an offering back to the Beloved, and out to all beings everywhere.

From this oceanic love consciousness, gently bring your awareness to the breath around your heart. Breathe softly into the tender space around your heart, your breath compassionately massaging and cradling it with its soft rhythm. Let your breath hold your heart lovingly, the way you would hold a baby. Rest here as long as you like.

From the vast spaciousness of *Savasana,* gradually let your breath begin to awaken you the way you would slowly and tenderly awaken a child. Notice how with the body so relaxed and receptive, the breath flows easily. When you feel ready to move, slowly roll to your right side, and rest there for a few more heartbeats. Experience the sweetness of simply resting on the earth, fully supported and held.

> In the morning when I began to wake,
> It happened again—
> That feeling, that You, Beloved, had stood over me all night
> Keeping watch.
> That feeling that as soon as I began to stir
> You put Your lips on my forehead
> And lit a Holy Lamp inside my heart.
>
> —HAFIZ[18]

Feeling that holy lamp lit inside your heart, slowly support yourself up into a sitting position, sitting with the awareness of the glowing light that you carry within. Sit so that your heart sun can freely radiate that sacred love out to all beings everywhere.

Sit quietly for a while and savor the holiness of embodying the light of love. Let your sitting posture express your wonder, gratitude, and boundless compassion. Bringing your hands to the Namaste position at the heart center, bow your head and dedicate your yoga practice to the benefit of all beings everywhere.

> May all beings be safe from inner and outer harm,
> May all beings be peaceful and happy,
> May all beings be healthy and strong,
> May all beings care for themselves joyfully,
> May all beings love themselves completely.
>
> —METTA PRAYER OF LOVING-KINDNESS

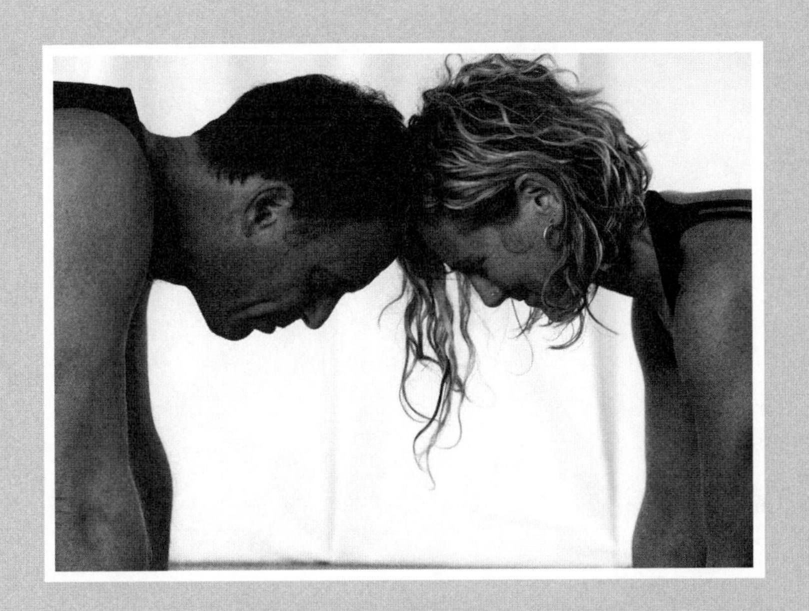

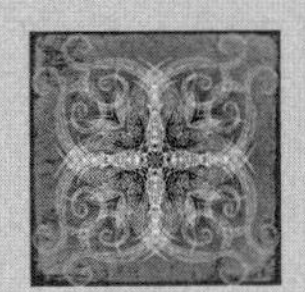 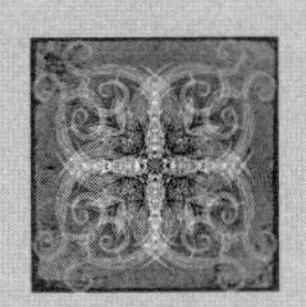 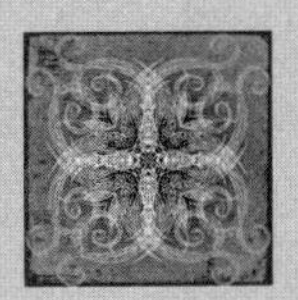

SEVEN
The Joy of Tantra

The word *"Tantra"* is derived from the Sanskrit *tan,* to stretch and expand. *"Tantric"* signifies those disciplines by which knowledge and consciousness are stretched and expanded, so that the full passion, power, and wisdom of the One can infuse and illuminate them and bring the individual into an all-embracing union with the divine.

The magnificent tradition of Tantra first made its literary appearance in Hinduism toward the middle of the first millennium CE. From the beginning, it celebrated the feminine aspect of the Godhead, the Shakti—the fire-energy that streams from the source to engender the creation and live in it. To the Tantric, the whole universe is the child of the Mother-Father. As the great Kalidasa wrote, "Everything that exists runs with the golden love juices of Shiva and Shakti, and is bathed in the perfumes that stream from their naked glory."

The great Tantric formula is Samsara equals Nirvana, which reveals that the world and the creation in all their holy particulars are co-essential with the transcendent *Sat/Chit/Ananda* or being/consciousness/bliss. Everything in its inherent bliss nature is divine and holy. There is nothing but God in us and around us at all times. For the Tantric, liberation (or enlightenment) does not come from renouncing reality, abandoning the world, or extinguishing the exuberance of one's natural desires. Rather, authentic freedom spontaneously arises when what has been categorized as "lower reality" is experienced as contained within and melting into the "higher." At the same time, this "higher reality" is constantly invoked to penetrate and transfigure the "lower," at ever-greater depths of power, presence, and rapture.

We shall be concentrating in Heart Yoga on what we call the Tantra of tenderness, a Tantra that allows us to use the body as an instrument of tender compassion toward all beings. However, we do not want to ignore the great and holy Tantra of liberated and consecrated sexuality. We believe that when it is practiced along with the Tantra of tenderness, it can provide human beings with an inexhaustible abundance of the energy and impassioned delight essential as a foundation for pouring ourselves out in loving service to the world.

Walt Whitman has perfectly expressed the revelation of a reality pervaded at all levels by ecstatic love that the Tantra of liberated, consecrated, and illumined love engenders.

> I believe in you my soul . . . the other I am must not abase itself
> to you,
> And you must not be abased to the other.
> Loafe with me on the grass . . . loose the stop from your throat,
> Not words, not music or rhyme I want . . . not custom or lecture, not
> even the best,
> Only the lull I like, the hum of your valued voice.
> I mind how we lay in June, such a transparent summer morning;
> You settled your head athwart my hips and gently turned over
> upon me,
> And parted the shirt from my bosom-bone, and plunged your tongue
> to my barestript heart,
> And reached till you felt my beard, and reached till you held my feet.
> Swiftly arose and spread around me the peace and joy and
> knowledge that pass all the art and argument of the earth;
> And I know that the hand of God is the elderhand of my own,
> And I know that the spirit of God is the eldest brother of my own,
> And that all the men ever born are also my brothers . . . and the
> women my sisters and lovers,
> And that a kelson of the creation is love;
> And limitless are leaves stiff or drooping in the fields,
> And brown ants in the little wells beneath them,
> And mossy scabs of the wormfence, and heaped stones, and elder
> and mullein and pokeweed.[1]

Everything that we have been trying to communicate in this book about the all-transforming peace of the Transcendent and its irradiation in love, of the Immanent, is transmitted here through a vision that arises from Tantric abandon, a vision that embraces not only the lover with whom Whitman shares his transparent summer ecstasy, but also all men and all women, "leaves stiff or drooping in the field," "brown ants," and even, most tenderly and miraculously, "elder and mullein and pokeweed." Every sense has, in the Tantric experience, found its most precise and divine intensity. Every realm of existence has been revealed as the subtle blazing of love.

A great anonymous Kabbalist of the thirteenth century wrote in the *Iggeret ha-Qodesh,*

> When sexual union is for the sake of heaven, there is nothing as holy or pure . . . thereby, one becomes a partner with God in the act of creation. This is the secret meaning of the saying of the sages: . . . when [two beings, devoted to each other in heart, mind, and body unite] "the divine presence is between them." Human thought has the power to expand and ascend to its origin. Attaining the source, she is joined with the upper light from which she emanated. She and he become one. Then when thought emanates once again, all become a single ray: the upper light is drawn down by the power of thought. In this way the divine presence appears on Earth. A bright light shines and spreads around the place where the meditator is sitting. Similarly, when [two devoted beings] unite, and their thought joins the beyond, that thought draws down the upper light.[2]

Another Kabbalist, Baruch ben Abraham, describes how, for years, he believed that a saying of the Torah, "one should hallow oneself during sexual union," meant that "One should sanctify one's thought by eliminating any intention of feeling physical pleasure." He adds, however, "Sometime later, God favored me with a gift of grace, granting me understanding of the essence of sexual holiness. The holiness derives precisely from feeling the pleasure. The secret is wondrous, deep and awesome."[3]

It is this "wondrous, deep, and awesome" secret that the Heart Yoga of the celebration of Tantra prays to make available to all human beings. For too many millennia, our separation from the sanctity of the Divine Feminine has divorced us from the wisdom and ecstatic health to be found in liberated desire. The world needs Tantric lovers now, lovers who use their Tantric experience as a way of entering, as Kalidasa, Whitman, and the Kabbalistic sages did, into the holy passion of the One for its creation, and of infusing their entire being with this holy passion so as to be able to serve the world tirelessly.

> Passion burns down every branch of exhaustion;
> Passion is the Supreme Elixir and renews all things;
> No one can grow exhausted when passion is born!
> Don't sigh heavily, your brow bleak with boredom;
> Look for passion, passion, passion, passion!
> . . . Run my friends, run far away from all false solutions!
> Let Divine Passion triumph and rebirth you in yourself!
>
> —RUMI, from the *Mathnawi*[4]

Yoga Practice Sequence to Celebrate the Joy of Tantra

- Cross-legged Sitting – *Sukhasana*
- Child's Pose – *Adho Mukha Virasana*
- Hands and Knees Pose
- Hands and Knees Pose with Partner
- Downward-facing Dog Pose – *Adho Mukha Svanasana*
- Downward-facing Dog Pose with Partner
- Child's Pose with Partner – *Adho Mukha Virasana*
- Standing Forward Bend – *Uttanasana*
- Mountain Pose – *Tadasana*
- Sun Salutation – *Surya Namaskar*
- Sun Salutation with Partner
- Mountain Pose – *Tadasana*

- Tree Pose – *Vrksasana*
- Seated Twist – *Bharadvajasana*
- Seated Twist with Partner
- Bound Angle Pose – *Baddha Konasana*
- Pelvic Rocking
- Restorative Rest
- *Savasana*

This sequence of yoga poses celebrates the Tantra of tenderness. It can be practiced alone or with a partner. These poses are designed to gently initiate you into the divine paradox at the heart of Tantra. It is necessary to first be grounded in your own body, and stabilized in a realization of the universal love energy that dances in and as all things. Only then, without fear or resistance, can you truly see, celebrate, and cherish another. The divine in you will recognize the divine in them, and effortless love will arise within you.

By bringing you into your own divine heart and luminous body, these poses will inspire you to extend unconditional love to others. This love, arising from the clearest and deepest aspect of your being, will soar free of the grasping mind which needs to define, possess, and control.

In the Tantra of tenderness, the divine in you loves and celebrates the divine appearing, in mystery and wonder, in others. As this experience deepens, you will come to know that you are living the love of the Divine itself. As Blake wrote, "eternity is in love with the productions of time."

When the eternal love consciousness in you marries the divine awareness of your body, you enter into union with the Mother-Father, and you love all beings directly as a manifestation of that union.

Through the practice of the Tantra of tenderness, you will taste the joy of divine love as pure offering and prayer. Whether you are alone or with another, the glowing diamond lamp of love radiates tenderly from you. Let the perfect marriage of peace and passion, body and soul that the *Song of Songs* transmits be your guide to this practice.

I am my beloved's
And he is mine.
Come, my beloved,
Let us go forth into the field
And lodge in the villages.
Let us go up early to the vineyards;
Let us see whether the vine hath budded,
Whether the grape hath opened,
And the pomegranates are in bloom.
There will I give thee my love.
The mandrakes give forth fragrance,
And at our doors are all manner of precious fruits, new and old,
Which I have laid up for thee, O my beloved.

—*Song of Songs* 7:10–13[5]

The poses in this section can be adapted to individual practice by using a wall or props. Practicing this sequence alone, you can observe your relationship with yourself, and awaken self-compassion. You may experience a feeling of releasing the back of your heart, reinhabiting your heart, and a deeper love for yourself and others.

Poses practiced with partners explore and celebrate union. They provide an intimate way of opening to another in body, mind, heart, and spirit. They invite you to experience the subtle and healing nuances of giving and receiving. In times of disconnection, these practices can awaken the loving energy of authentic union, beyond personality issues and power struggle, and provide a healing container to observe these issues without judgment or resistance. They help you remember the love that is the true nature of your heart.

The word "yoga" comes from the Sanskrit word *yuj,* which means "yoke," or "union." In the Tantra of tenderness, allow the yoga to carry you into the depths of the mystery of relationship and union.

I honor the God and the Goddess,
The eternal parents of the universe.

The Lover, out of boundless love,
takes the form of the Beloved.
What beauty!
Both are made of the same nectar
and share the same food.

Out of Supreme Love
they swallow each other up,
But separate again
For the joy of being two.

They are not completely the same
But neither are they different.
None can tell exactly what they are.

How intense is their longing
To be with each other.
This is their greatest bliss.
Never, even in jest,

Do they allow their unity
to be disturbed.

They are so averse to separation
That even though they have become
This entire world,
Never for a moment do they let a difference
Come between them.

They sit together
On the same ground,
Both wearing a garment of light.

From the beginning of time
  They have been together,
Reveling in their own Supreme Love.

The difference they created
  To enjoy this world
Had one glimpse of their intimacy
And could not help
  But merge back into the bliss
  Found in their union.

Without the God
  There is no Goddess,
And without the Goddess
  There is no God.

How sweet is their love!
The entire universe
  Is too small to contain them,
Yet they live happily
  In the tiniest particle…
  —JNANESHWAR[6]

Cross-Legged Sitting
Sukhasana
With a partner:

Sit facing each other, and light a candle between you. See each other in the light of tenderness, through the eyes of your heart. Silently gaze at each other, seeing beyond words and thoughts into the essence of the being in front of you.

Hold hands, or place your hands on each other's hearts. Bless each other, either silently or with a few heart-felt words. Draw your hands to your heart in the Namaste position of prayer, and bow reverently to each other.

Remember that *namaste* can be translated as "The divine light within me salutes the divine light within you." When you feel yourself filled with respect and love for the other, as well as for yourself, move into Child's Pose, absorbing the tender awakening of your heart into the depths of every cell.

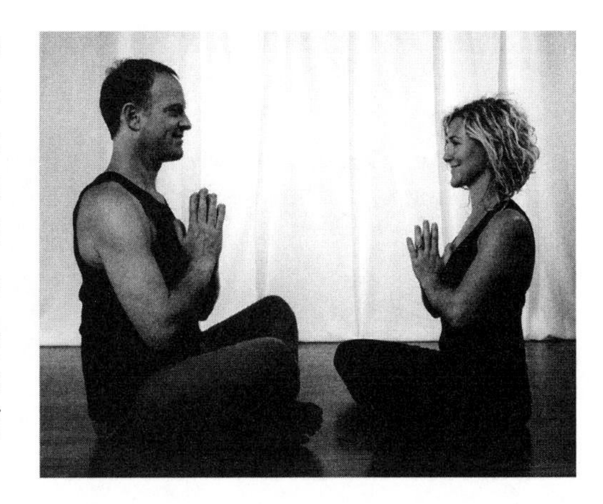

Individual practice:

Sit comfortably, with your spine erect. Light a candle, and attune yourself to how you're feeling in this precious moment. Krishnamurti states that observation without judgment is the highest form of spiritual practice. Inwardly gaze at yourself without judgment. See yourself with compassion, kindness, and mercy, as if you were looking at yourself through the eyes of the Mother, the Buddha, or Christ. You may wish to repeat to yourself the following Buddhist loving-kindness prayer:

> May I be free from inner and outer harm.
> May I be happy and peaceful.
> May I be healthy and strong.
> May I care for myself joyfully.

Child's Pose

Adho Mukha Virasana

Come to a kneeling position, slightly widening your knees. If you are practicing with a partner, kneel facing each other, about six feet apart. Sink your feet, shins, and thighs down into the earth while gently lifting your belly and heart. With an exhalation, slowly release your chest onto your thighs, resting your hands by your feet, palms soft like a baby's hands.

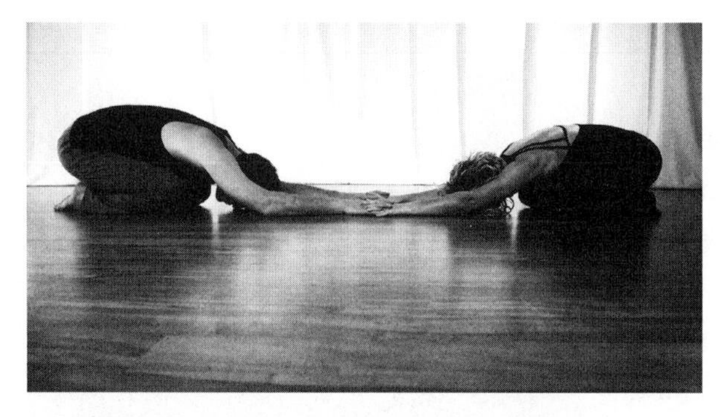

Rest your forehead on your mat or on a bolster, curled in the position of the embryo.

Rest in this position of prayer, melting into the strong loving arms of Mother Earth. Notice how your breath naturally flows into the backs of your lungs, opening your back ribs like feathers, while your kidneys widen and release. Reach out your hands in front of you, toward your partner, touching each other's hands.

Let your back body open now like spreading wings, lifting you into the spaciousness of Father Sky around and above you. With each breath, open every cell to the blessing of the marriage of the Mother's tenderness and nurturance rising in warm energy from the earth, and the blessing of the Father's infinite protection raining down upon you as light-energy from above.

In Child's Pose, we open our outer body to receive the protective blessing of the Father while surrendering our inner body to the nurturing tenderness of the Mother. We can experience in our bodies, as the great mystic Ramakrishna, paraphrasing Kabir said, that "The formless absolute is my Father, and God with form is my Mother."[7] In Child's Pose, we incarnate and birth the sacred marriage of form and formlessness, the Mother-Father. Experiencing this, our whole being can become infused with tenderness toward all life.

Hands and Knees Pose

(with pubic bone/tailbone awareness)

Child's Pose prepares you to begin the experience of the Sacred Marriage within your body. After a few minutes in this position, follow the holy and sensual exploration of the dance of the pubic bone and tailbone as it leads you deeper into the mystery of the union of the Mother-Father within your body.

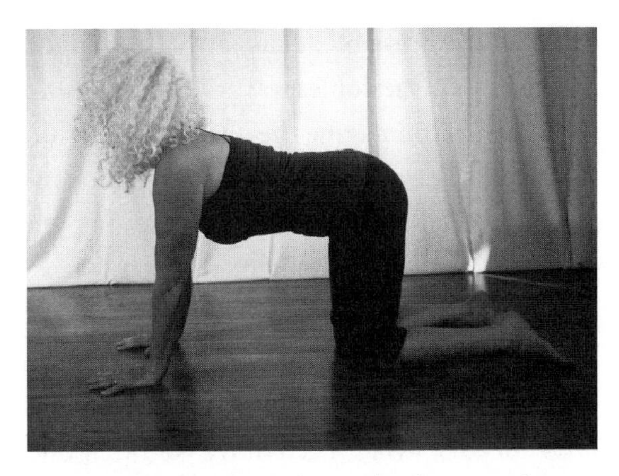

Come to your hands and knees and feel your roots dropping into the earth. Watch how your breath naturally moves your body. Approach this practice with reverence, for it can take you deep into the erotic radiance of the marriage of the Mother-Father in the cells of your body. Trust the wisdom and intuition of your body to guide you to create your own authentic practice. The more aware you are of the subtle nuances of this practice, the more it will reveal to you.

On your inhalation, your sacrum, the sacred bone, tips forward, while with your exhalation your tailbone descends. There is a very subtle rocking through the basin of your pelvis with each breath. Let the breath be a lamp guiding you deep inside your body, helping you to focus on this gentle movement with loving attention.

With every inhalation your pubic bone is attracted toward your tailbone, like iron filings drawn toward a magnet. With each exhalation your tailbone is also magnetically drawn toward your pubic bone. As your pubic bone moves toward your tailbone on the inhalation, let your whole front body release.

Continue slowly back and forth, becoming aware of the connection between all twenty-six of your vertebrae. Initiated from the movement of your watery flowing pelvis, the vertebrae ripple up and down. As your pelvis releases, a wave pulses throughout your spine.

Richard Freeman, a brilliant yoga teacher awake to the subtle mystical dimensions of yoga, offers an exquisite analogy for the dance of the pubic bone and tailbone.[8] He invites us to imagine that the pubic bone is the queen, the divine feminine, and the front of the body is the queen's royal temple filled with her priestesses. On the inhalation, the priestesses accompany the queen in a procession as she moves toward the king, the tailbone, the divine masculine. As she comes toward him, the king backs away. Richard Freeman then asks us to imagine the back body as the king's royal temple containing his priests. They accompany the king, the tailbone, as he moves on the exhalation toward the queen. She responds by backing away. The front body opens, then the back body opens, in a softly rocking sensual rhythm led by the breath.

Begin to make this movement even smaller and subtler. Allow your pubic bone to move toward your tailbone, while your tailbone stays stable and does not back away. Then move your tailbone toward your pubic bone while the pubic bone stays stable and does not retreat. As the movement between your pubic bone and your tailbone becomes subtler and smaller, you will notice that the vibration between them becomes stronger, just as a pot lid dropped on the floor spins and vibrates faster and faster before it becomes still again.

Feel how your tailbone and pubic bone are irresistibly drawn toward each other. Experience their longing to unite in the marriage bed between them. This mysterious bed, the perineum, domes up into your body as your pubic bone and tailbone vibrate toward each other. Root your awareness in this velvety marriage bed, and from there, spread its softly quivering energy evenly throughout your body.

Glorious is the moment we sit in the palace, you and I
Two forms, two faces, but a single soul, you and I
The flowers will blaze and bird cries shower us with immortality
The moment we enter the garden, you and I
All the stars of heaven will run out to gaze at us
As we burn as the full moon itself, you and I
The fire-winged birds of heaven will rage with envy
In that place we laugh ecstatically, you and I
What a miracle, you and I, entwined in the same nest
What a miracle, you and I, one love, one lover, one Fire

In this world and the next, in an ecstasy without end.
—RUMI[9]

The pubic bone/tailbone dance is similar to the dance of relationship. In relationship counseling, this interaction is called the dance of the pursuer and the distancer. When the pursuing partner comes forward, the distancing one moves backward. They keep an unconsciously agreed-upon space between them.

When you stay firm in your tailbone but draw your pubic bone toward it, allowing your tailbone to receive the pubic bone, and when you widen your pubic bone and allow the tailbone to be received by the pubic bone, then the space between the two bones becomes luminously charged. These bones move toward each other in the magical space of the perineum. The perineum is the marriage bed of the body, the root known as the *muladhara* chakra.

As you consciously draw the pubic bone and tailbone toward each other, the subtle energy of the gateway of the root chakra, known as *mula bandha,* is awakened, and energy effortlessly flows upward, flooding the whole body-mind.

This energy may feel like a burst of primordial, solar energy within the body. It is from this sacred solar fire that sexuality, Tantric tenderness, and the kundalini energy arise. Bring this sensuously vibrating energy into the yoga practice of the Tantra of tenderness, suffusing all the poses with its awakened power.

Hands and Knees Pose with Partner

Remain in the Hands and Knees Pose, facing each other. Press the crown of your head into the crown of your partner's head. Gently move your head up and down, side to side, in circles, or in any spontaneous movement, always keeping your head joined to your partner's head. One partner might push while the other recedes, and then roles will reverse. See what happens naturally, enjoying the playfulness of this connection.

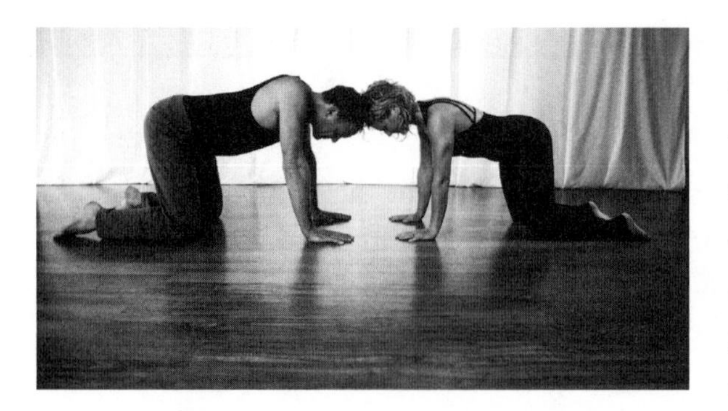

Gradually slow down the movement and return to the original position, simply feeling your heads opening to each other. Stay for a while in stillness, and then very slowly draw away from each other, noticing the electro-magnetic energy that longs to hold you in this sacred union. Feel the energy vibrating through your body from your tailbone to the crown of your head.

Downward-facing Dog Pose
Adho Mukha Svanasana
(with partner or alone)

Keep your awareness in the deep, velvety chamber of the marriage bed of your body (the perineum area), as well as in the crown center. From your hands and knees, lift up into Dog Pose by floating your belly up, releasing your tailbone toward the sky. Bend your legs and again find the same vibrant rocking movement between your pubic bone and tailbone. Inhale, and surrender the pubic bone toward your tailbone, curling your tailbone up as if you were one of those dogs with the really curly tails that curl back toward their head. Exhale, and as your belly empties, invite your tailbone toward your widening pubic bone.

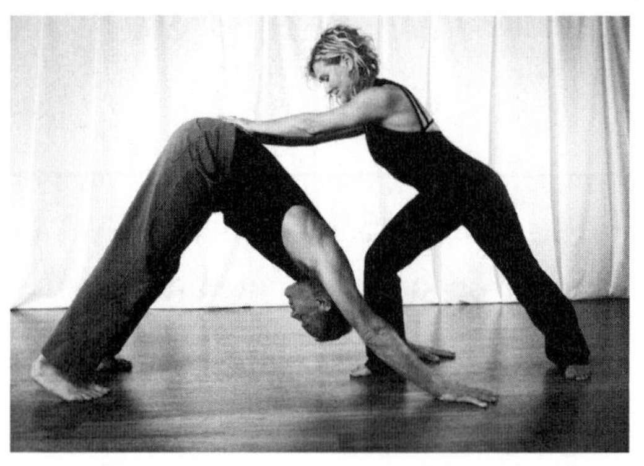

Rock for a few breaths, and then slow down the outer movement until it becomes a subtle inner vibration. From the pelvis, move your legs back and steady them, and lengthen your arms. Again from the root chakra, the source of this luminous, vibrating aliveness, spread energy evenly from the marriage bed root to every cell in your body.

Rest in Child's Pose when you become tired, then rise up once again into Dog Pose. Keep unfolding into Dog Pose, lifting your hips while moving down through the roots of your hands and feet. Let your head drop. Lift from the arches of your feet, and also from the arch between your tailbone and pubic bone, so that the energy from Mother Earth can stream into your body and fill it evenly and fully. Breathe it in, and with the exhalation radiate it outward into the world. Stay as long as you wish, then return to Child's Pose.

Downward-facing Dog Pose with Partner

If you are practicing with a partner, you can adjust each other in Dog Pose in the following way. First simply observe your partner in Dog Pose, seeing them with tenderness and compassion. Stand by their hands, and put the heels of your hands just under the top of their sacrum at the top of their buttocks. Lean forward onto your hands, using your weight to draw their sacrum up toward their sitting bones. Notice how their spine elongates. Stay here for a few breaths, and then slowly release your hands from their back. The partner in Dog Pose stays for a while, feeling the lightness in their body from their partner's support, then slowly releases into Child's Pose.

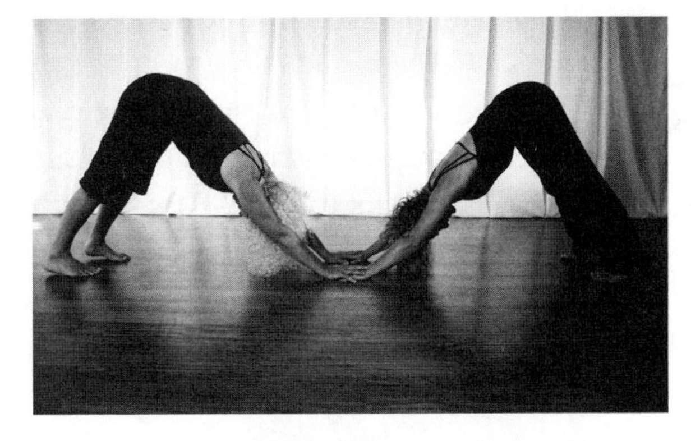

Child's Pose with Partner

To adjust your partner in Child's Pose, stand over their head and place your hands on at the top of their pelvis. Draw their buttocks down toward their sitting bones, as you did in Dog Pose. This helps them to lengthen their back and release their hips. They will probably enjoy quite a strong touch, so you can

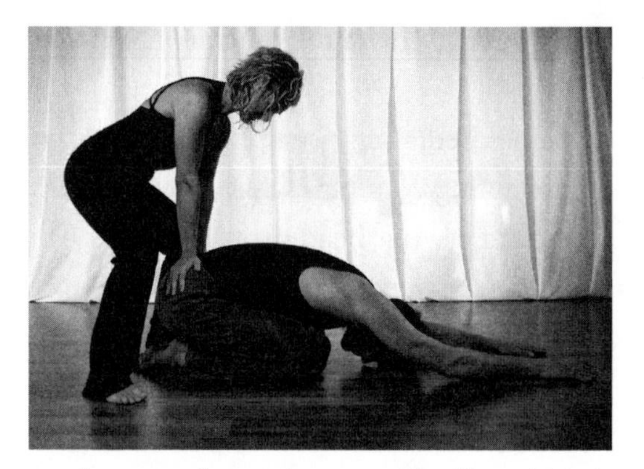

use your body weight to press the buttocks down toward their heels. Be sure you both communicate about how much pressure is appropriate. After five or six breaths, walk your hands up either side of their spine, massaging their back as you do so. Let your hands express the tenderness of your heart, and offer a blessing for your partner's well-being.

Standing Forward Bend
Uttanasana
(with partner or alone)

Return to Dog Pose for a few breaths, facing your partner or on your own, then step both feet forward and place your hands on your thighs. Again, gently rock your pelvis. With your inhalation your chest and head lift. With your exhalation your belly floats toward your heart and head, and your back body opens and rounds. Inhale, and create a slight backbend, your head receiving the action from your pelvis. Exhale, and feel your pelvis dropping back, your tailbone descending, your belly surging up toward your heart, and your head emptying.

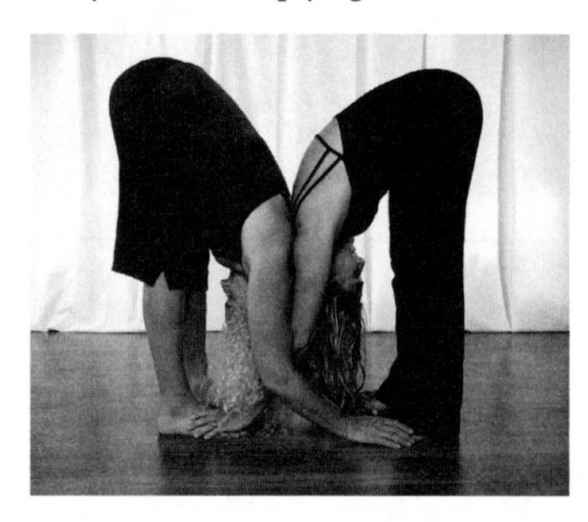

Inhale and lift your collarbones; exhale and lift your belly and drop your head. With the inhalation, your groin deepens and softens back. With the exhalation, the wings of your kidneys lift and spread, and your head empties. If you are practicing with a partner, experiment with leaning your backs into each other for support. With your next exhalation, let your belly float up lightly like a helium balloon through the center of your body. Separate your backs and roll up through your spine, spreading the wings of your arms above you. Come up to a gentle standing backbend for a few breaths, and then bring your hands to your heart, softening your eyes and bowing to your partner or yourself.

Mountain Pose

Tadasana

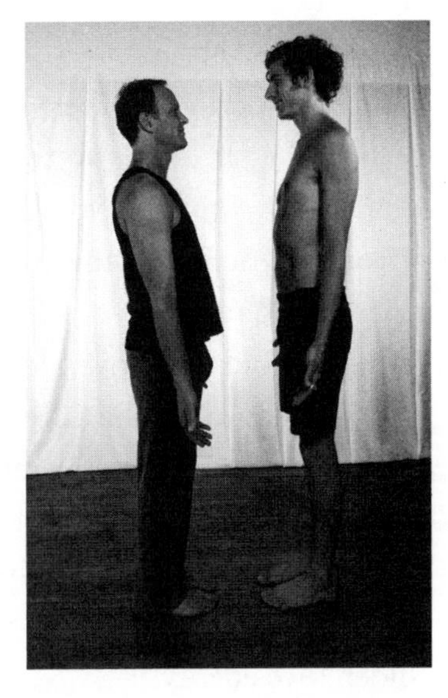

Come to a standing position. In Mountain Pose for the Tantra of tenderness practice, we again experience the fluid dancing Tantric energy of the pelvis, combined with the stability of the mountain. Bring your hands to your pelvis, one hand to your belly, one hand to the back of your sacrum. Feel the slight pelvic rocking movement with your breath, like the fiery core breathing inside a volcano. Sense the sacred energy that you are holding between your hands. With your inhalation, let your pelvis tip forward a bit and your pubic bone drop away from your navel. With your exhalation, your belly empties and floats up into your heart.

As you inhale, imagine your breath descending into your heart. As you exhale, imagine your breath floating up through the top of your head, like a whale's breath. Inhale down through your groin and feet into the earth. Exhale out the top of your head like a fountain releasing into the sky. Your body becomes a channel between earth with your inhalation and sky with your exhalation.

The wave of your breath flows through your body evenly in *Tadasana*. Within the majestic steadiness of Mountain Pose, feel how your body is vibrating and pulsing with aliveness.

Sun Salutation

Surya Namaskar

Stand in Mountain Pose, drawing your hands together in front of your heart in the Namaste position. Bow your head slightly and feel your mind sink into the bed of your heart. Salute the divine light within you and all around you.

Sweep your arms out to the sides like wings opening from your heart, outlining the auric circle of divine light enfolding you. Bring your hands together above you and draw this light down into your body, through the thousand-petaled lotus of the crown chakra, through the diamond clarity at the third eye, through the soft red petals of the throat, into the shining golden chalice of your heart. Feel your heart burn softly in the fire of divine love.

Empty your hands so that they can be open channels of heart energy. Again, let the wings of your heart sweep open, describing the light-body that surrounds you. Sense the aura radiating out from your center like a golden sphere of light.

Exhale and bend over, leading from your heart and hinging from your hips. You can bend the knees here to make it easy and gentle. Touching the earth in gratitude and reverence, drop your head. Slide one foot back, still feeling the stability of the feet and the legs on earth, and then the other foot back. Release your knees, chest, and chin to the floor, placing your hands under your shoulders. Sweep your heart up, radiating from it a flow of warm golden love energy.

Come to Sphinx Pose with your elbows and hands on the floor. Rock from leg to leg, and then draw them together. Your legs hug the mid-line of your body, melting into each other until they feel like a broad kangaroo tail. Press that tail down into the earth, and allow your heart to respond by lifting and offering itself in love.

Sweep back to Child's Pose. Breathe deeply, releasing your body to the earth. Come to your hands and knees, curl your toes under, and lift up to Dog Pose, dropping your head. Awaken all the cells in your body to the fire of love that is growing in you. As Rumi wrote,

How can you ever hope to know the Beloved
Without becoming in every cell the Lover?

Step forward from Dog Pose to the Standing Forward Bend pose. Exhale, letting your head drop, and scoop up through your belly. Spread the wings of your arms from your heart, honoring all beings. Draw awareness into your heart center as you return your hands to your heart in the prayer position.

Sense the energy ascending from Mother Earth through your lower body and descending from Father Sky through your upper body. Marry earth and sky in the sacred temple of your heart.

Sun Salutation with Partner
Surya Namaskar

Stand in Mountain Pose, facing your partner about four feet apart. Salute the divine light within both you and your partner. Slowly move through another *Surya Namaskar,* the salutation to the sun, honoring the divine sun you see reflected in your partner. You can experiment with mirroring each other's movements, or move at your own rhythm.

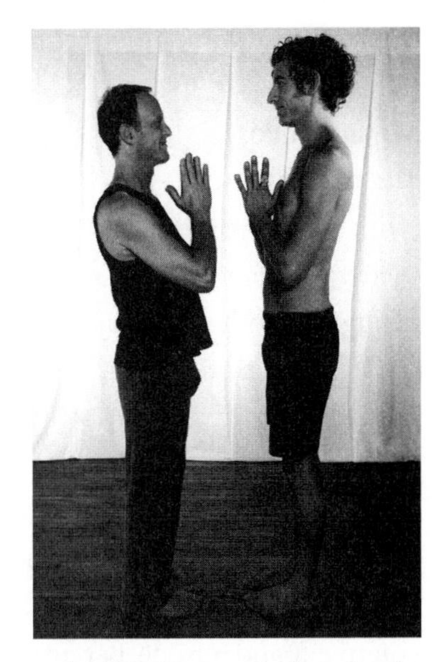

Inhale, and as you sweep your arms up draw a circle of golden light around you and your partner. Consciously embrace and contain your partner within that sphere of light. Exhale and bow to each other, bending your knees if you like, and touch the earth with your hands. Step one foot back, then the other. You can release your knees to the floor or take your body down toward the floor all at once, moving slowly and mindfully. Curling up into an easy Cobra Pose, let your heart radiate forward in love toward your partner. Come to your hands and knees and lift into Dog Pose, bowing to each other and lengthening your spine. Step forward again, coming into the Lunge Pose (page 69), offering your heart energy to your partner while remaining firmly grounded in yourself. Step forward with the other foot, coming into the Forward Bend.

Lift through the arches of your feet while embedding the soles firmly into Mother Earth. Lift up through the floor of your pelvis, and spread your arms wide as you roll up to standing. With open arms, send love and gratitude to your partner, embracing him or her with your heart energy. Let your body express the depth of tenderness you feel for your partner. Open and receive in your body, mind, and heart the gift of love sent from your partner.

Bringing your hands to the prayer position, bow to your partner, and pray silently that your relationship will continue to be illumined by the tenderness you are experiencing in this practice. Notice the difference in practicing Sun Salutation alone and with a partner.

Mountain Pose
Tadasana
(with partner or alone)

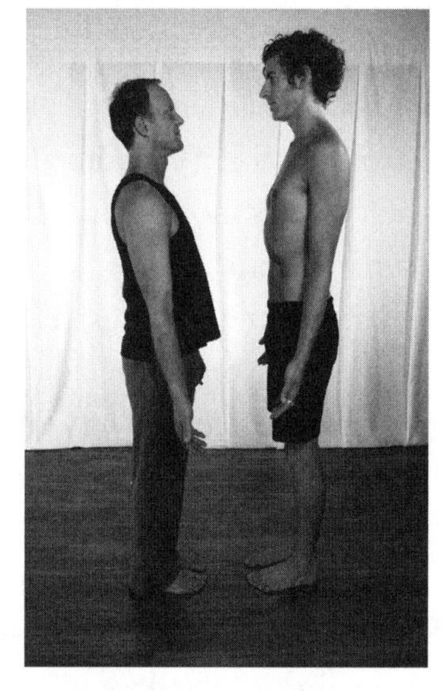

If you are practicing with a partner, stand facing each other. If you are practicing alone, consider facing a mirror, becoming your own partner.

In this *Tadasana*, grounded in your true essence, you uncover the courage to open and expose your whole being to your partner. Standing within the depths of yourself allows you to expand into deeper and deeper feelings of love for your partner. Give and receive the gift of pure loving presence. As you stand facing each other, be alert to any fear or vulnerability that may arise. Gently explore whatever you meet with acceptance and loving curiosity, as a guide from beyond.

This being human is a guest house.
Every morning a new arrival.

A joy, a depression, a meanness,
some momentary awareness comes
as an unexpected visitor.

Welcome and entertain them all!
Even if they're a crowd of sorrows,
Who violently sweep your house
empty of its furniture,
still, treat each guest honorably.
He may be clearing you out
for some new delight.

The dark thought, the shame, the malice,
meet them at the door laughing
and invite them in.

Be grateful for whoever comes,
because each has been sent
as a guide from beyond.

—RUMI[10]

Spread your feet to receive the energy from the earth beneath you. Invite your feet to open by lifting your toes off the floor and widening them so you can feel the air between every toe. Draw your big toes together and place them down. Move your little toes to the outside, and spread the middle toes wide as they return to the floor. Feel your feet fully receiving the earth.

Move your weight forward slightly to the front of your feet and lift your heels up. Then draw the fronts of the heels back as you lower them, opening your arches. Feel the round cushion of the heel embedded in the earth as if you were standing in mud, firmly rooted in the moist, warm earth.

Sense the earth energy flowing up through the channels of your legs. Bring your hands to the tops of your thighbones and gently guide them back behind you, so that they move back within your legs and your legs feel firmly rooted. Your heart lifts and expands, and your legs become as stable as a mountain.

With your inhalation, your pubic bone is again drawn toward your tailbone, as your sitting bones move back. Your tailbone descends like a huge taproot into the earth and meets the movement of the pubic bone. From the mysterious marriage between your tailbone and pubic bone, light flows up the front of the spine into the watery pelvis.

Breathing into your belly, allow it to soften so that this light-energy can flow through like water. The belly is like a vast ocean; let it spread out to all the bony landmarks of your pelvis. Silently, from the centered, grounded stability of *Tadasana,* offer a prayer for the peace and liberation of your partner and all beings.

Tree Pose
Vrksasana
(with a partner or alone)

If you are practicing alone, explore practicing in front of a mirror, or with the support of a wall. If you are practicing Tree Pose with a partner, first create your own stability and then play with the dance of energy that flows back and forth between you as you lovingly support and balance each other. In some forests, all the trees share a common root system. The forest looks like it is composed of separate trees, but actually all the roots are so intertwined that you can't separate them. In Tree Pose with a partner, imagine your roots uniting in this way, so that you feel that you are both growing from a common source.

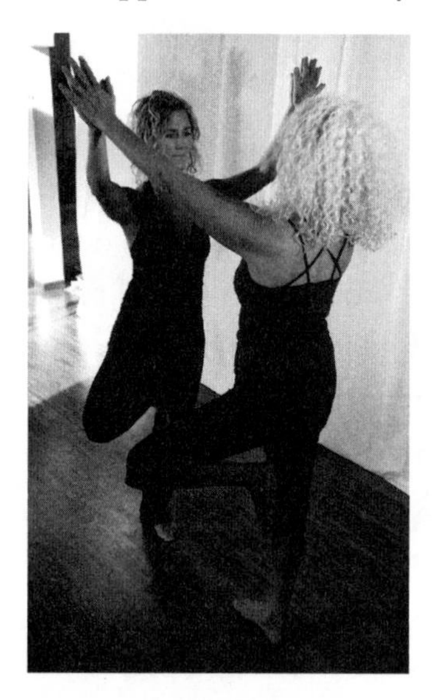

Bring the stability of *Tadasana,* the Mountain Pose, into *Vrksasana,* the Tree Pose. Begin by opening your feet, sending your roots deep into the earth. If you're practicing with a partner, notice how your roots become intermingled and undistinguishable in the darkness of the earth below. Draw up from this vast network of roots and let energy rise through the arches of your feet and up through the channel of your legs.

Shift your weight to your left leg, turning your right leg out. Bend your right knee and place the sole of your right foot against the inside of your left thigh. Point your right foot down, at the center of your inner thigh. Bring your hands to your heart, bow to your partner, and then release your arms above your head, palms facing each other. Send your roots down and feel the rebounding energy through the core channel of your body like sap rising. Sense the protection of Father Sky, meeting the nourishment of Mother Earth in the core of your being.

Keep your eyes soft, your jaw relaxed, your skin open, and your hands awake. Open your peripheral vision to see all around you, and sense your partner practicing near you. Notice, as your tailbone and pubic bone move toward each other, how energy surges up through your trunk and your belly lifts toward the back of your diaphragm, lifting heart energy up into the spaciousness of your head. Feel your body become a channel between the earth and the sky. Send your roots down, feeling the sap rising up within the container of the bark of your skin.

From your core, reach the branches of your arms out to touch your partner's branches, and feel how your branches can dance together, swaying in the wind. Press your hands together to support each other's balance.

When both of you are ready, steadily and slowly return to *Tadasana.* Place your foot down consciously just like a bird landing lightly in its nest. Feel the stability and balance of standing on your two feet.

Repeat Tree Pose to the other side. Again lift your heart and your branches and press your hands into each other's hands. If practicing alone, you can press your hands into the support of a wall. Explore separating your hands from each other or from the wall, and notice how different Tree Pose feels without outer support.

Feel the warmth and touch of your partner's hands and the energy that flows through their hands into yours, and from your hands into their hands. Lift your heart in celebration of your love for one another. Notice the ease of balance when love supports form, and when the illusion of separateness begins to dissolve.

Keeping your hands connected and hearts lifting, slowly lower your hands so that your arms can rest, keeping your connection as you come back to *Tadasana.* Stand in the Mountain Pose, not as a separate mountain, but as two interconnecting mountains, merging into one. Slowly release your hands from your partner's, yet feel how united you remain. Close your eyes for a few breaths, noticing how you feel now in *Tadasana.* Return to the root of yourself. Allow the love and connection you've experienced to flood and illumine your relationship.

> Blessed are those who trust in the Lord,
> Whose trust is in the Lord.
> They shall be like a tree planted by water,
> Sending out its roots by a stream.
> It shall not fear when heat comes,
> And its leaves shall stay green;
> In the year of drought it is not anxious,
> And does not cease to bear fruit.
>
> —JEREMIAH[11]

Seated Twist

Bharadvajasana

Sit on the floor with your legs outstretched. If you are practicing with a partner, sit facing each other, connecting the soles of your feet. Bend your legs and draw them to the left, placing your feet next to your left hip, and resting your right ankle on the arch of your left foot. You can place a small support under your right sitting bone to keep your pelvis level. Awaken your feet, and draw energy up your legs into your pelvis. Scoop up through

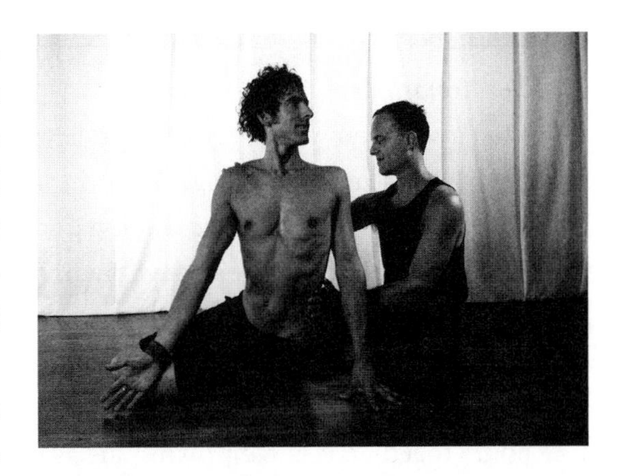

your belly, lifting your heart. Inhale, and lengthen from your tailbone to the crown of your head. Exhale, and begin releasing from your belly toward the right, continuing to root your feet and legs into the floor.

Root, rise, and release with each breath. With each exhalation, turn from the belly, ribs, shoulders, allowing your neck and head to gently receive the twist. Place your right hand behind you and move down through your fingers. Rest your left hand lightly on the outside of your right thigh. Move back through the left thigh and forward from the right hip to right knee, widening the thighs slightly like the blades of a pair of scissors opening. Feel energy spiraling up your spine. Stay at least five breaths and slowly return to center, resting for a few breaths with legs outstretched before releasing to the other side.

Seated Twist with Partner

One partner comes to the Seated Twist, and the other is the witness. As the witness you first simply sit and observe, seeing your partner with tenderness and compassion, through the eyes of your heart. Then exhale, sending heart energy into your hands, and lightly place your hands on your partner's kidneys just above their waist. Feel how their kidneys relax into the support of your hands. Follow the releasing of your partner's body as he or she turns more deeply into the twist, guided by the tender encouragement of your hands.

Intuitively spiral your hands up your partner's back, moving with their breath. With the gentle touch of your hands, invite your partner to explore the twist. Lightly touch the crown of the head, blessing them, and drawing loving energy up through the crown chakra. Repeat on the other side, and then trade places. Observe how you feel as a "giver" and as a "receiver."

Bound Angle Pose
Baddha Konasana
Sit facing away from your partner, hips elevated on a folded blanket or cushion, and spines almost touching. Draw the soles of your feet together. Inhale, softening your eyes. Exhale, expanding and emptying into the spaciousness around you. Remain here for a few breaths.

Staying with your inner focus, move back to back with your partner so that your spines are connected as intimately as possible. Draw the lowest point of your spines together at the tailbone, pressing your sacrum and sitting bones together. Feel your own spine as well as the warm support of your partner's spine, and the tender dialog between them. Melt your spines together, noticing how comfortable this pose is with the support of a partner.

If you're practicing alone, sit back against a wall, enjoying its support. If you're with a partner, experiment with releasing your hands behind you and resting them lightly on your partner's thighs. Allow your breathing to synchronize, letting your breath merge into one breath. When you're ready to part, do so slowly, feeling how hesitantly your backs peel away from each other. Sit for a few more breaths in Bound angle Pose, and notice how you feel without the physical support of your partner.

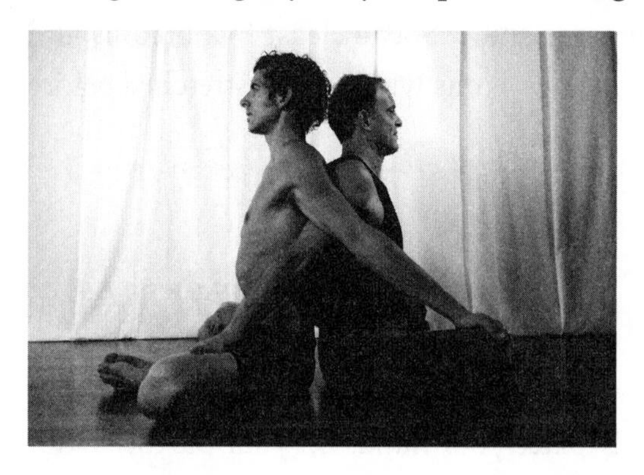

Pelvic Rocking
Slowly roll onto your back, bending your knees and coming onto your elbows. Place your hands under your kidneys, feeling them release into your hands. Slowly lengthen your spine away from your pelvis while sliding your hands down your hips to lengthen the skin of the buttocks toward the sitting bones. Rock tenderly from side to side, feeling the width of the sacrum as you release down onto the floor. Feel the sacrum supported on the floor.

Return to the experience of your tailbone moving to your pubic bone and your pubic bone moving to your tailbone. Feel the vibration between those two bones, and the doming up of the parachute of the perineum between them. Feel how the belly empties with the exhalation and releases to the back of the diaphragm. Then the light-flower of the heart opens, wafting its subtle fragrant light into the airiness inside the skull. Allow the motion of the pelvic rocking to slowly subside. Rest in the peace of this position.

Restorative Rest

(with partner)

Let your partner remain in the pelvic rocking position while you stand by their feet. Notice the angle of their thighs and bring your arms into the same line, placing your hands on your partner's knees. Lean your weight down through your arms, into their thighbones and into the sacrum. Notice their face relaxing and their breath deepening as their sacrum releases. Stay for about a minute, then gradually lift your hands away. Exchange roles, noticing how it feels to give, and how it feels to receive.

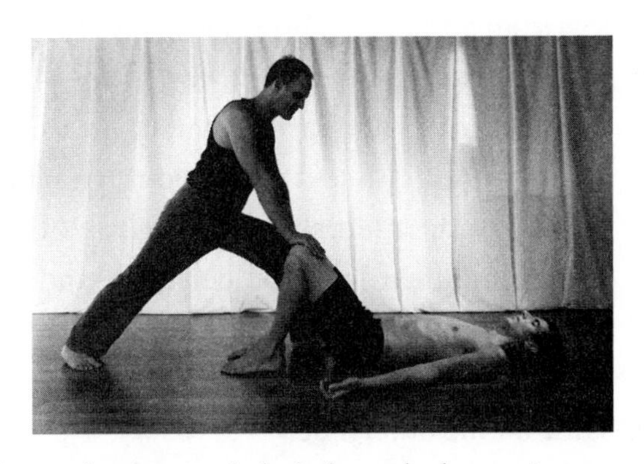

Turn to face your partner, bring your hands to the Namaste position, and let the divine in you bow to the divine in them.

Savasana

(with partner)

Bringing your partner into *Savasana* is an exquisitely tender gift for both of you. As you guide your partner into this position, allow the love you feel for him or her to flow from your heart out through your hands with each loving touch.

Let your partner lie back in *Savasana,* and sit by their feet. Feel their sweet

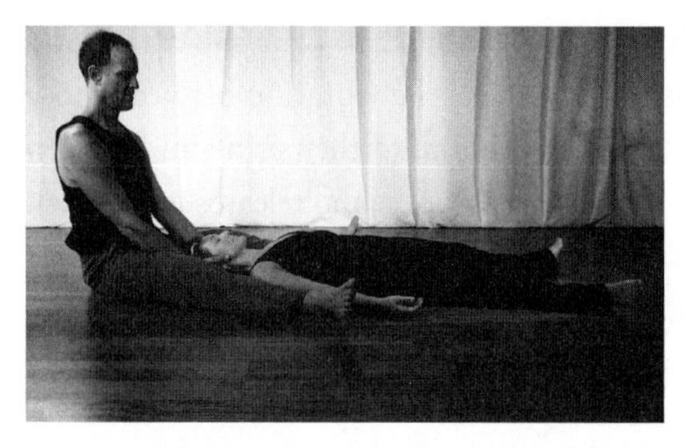

vulnerability, and your compassion. Cup their heels in your hands, and draw their legs toward you. Lift their legs slightly off the floor, and gently move the legs up and down a few times, feeling the thighbones release from the hips. Place their feet back onto the floor and massage them tenderly. Then stand over your partner, and one leg at a time sweep your hands down their legs from hips to feet, brushing away any tension. You can slide a rolled blanket or bolster under their knees.

Stand over your partner with your feet on either side of the hips, gazing at him or her with love. With your left hand crossing over their body, draw the top of their left shoulder slightly off the floor. Bring your right hand underneath their left shoulder blade and draw it down toward their waist. Roll the top of their shoulder down to the floor, and turn their left arm out. Sweep your hands down their arms and out through their fingers. Do the same on the other side.

Now sit by your partner's head and cradle it in your hands. Move your fingers under the ridge at the base of the skull and wait for the weight of the head to release into your hands. Draw their head toward you, lengthening their spine as you do so.

Sweep your hands along the skull and through your partner's hair. Place an eye pillow over their eyes and tenderly cover them with a blanket, as if you were tucking a child into bed.

Bless them with the sweet deep love you feel. You may wish to send them your heart energy with the Buddhist loving-kindness prayer:

> May you be safe from inner and outer harm.
> May you be happy and peaceful.

May you be healthy and strong.
May you care for yourself joyfully.

Savasana
(individual practice)

From the Restorative Rest Pose, slowly lengthen your feet to the floor. Sweep your consciousness over your body, releasing any tension. Allow the inside of your face to soften, your jaw to release, and the root of your tongue to relax. Your eyes drop within to gaze at your heart.

Feel yourself releasing back into the ocean of love consciousness. Let go for now of any holding, and settle back into yourself, like coming back home. Open yourself fully in this *Savasana* to the sweet tenderness inside you, and let yourself rest there, as long as you wish. (See page 52 for more detailed instructions regarding *Savasana*.)

So the sea-journey goes on, and who knows where!
Just to be held by the ocean is the best luck
we could have. It's a total waking up!
Why should we grieve that we've been sleeping?
It doesn't matter how long we've been unconscious.
We're groggy, but let the guilt go.
Feel the motions of tenderness
Around you, the buoyancy.

—RUMI[12]

When you're ready to return from *Savasana,* follow the current of your breath back to the ocean of your body. Feel how your breath rocks and cradles you as you rest on the motions of tenderness beneath you, fully supported. Slowly allow your breath to awaken you fully into this precious moment, awakening yourself as if you were awakening a child, with deep tenderness.

When you feel fully present, slowly roll to your right side, allowing your eyelids to part gradually. Return to yourself with compassion and love. When you are ready, come up to a sitting position. Sit for a while, savoring the peace of *Savasana*. Bow to the divine within you and all beings.

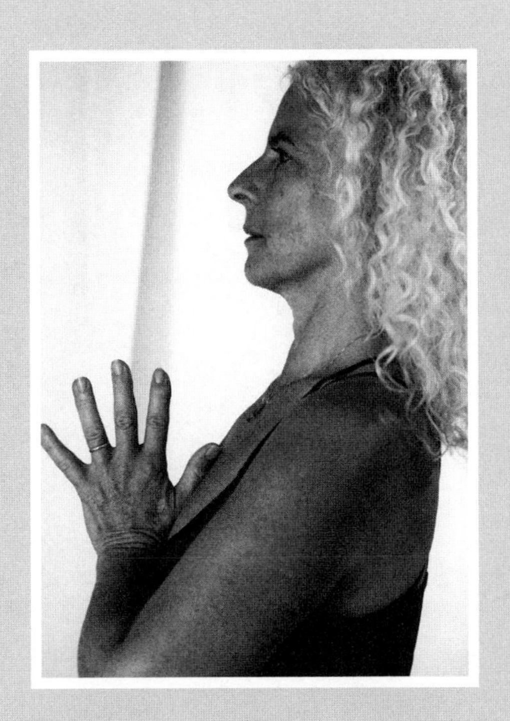

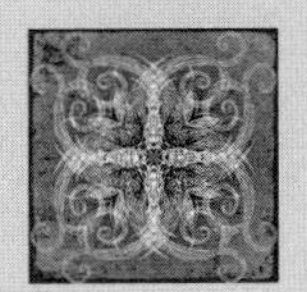 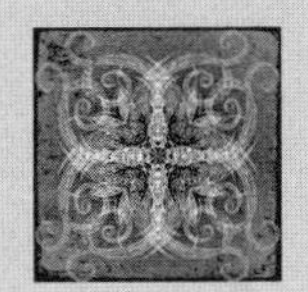 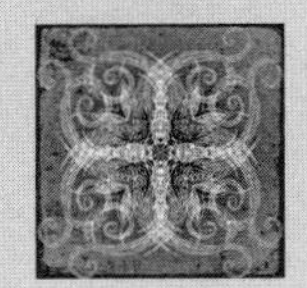

EIGHT
The Joy of Service

The finest human beings are those who constantly help others. The only master is the one who is the servant of his people. In the Koran it is written: "Never oppress the orphan. Never push away the beggar." To be just for one hour is worth more than praying for sixty years.

—RUMI[1]

Study is not the goal, doing is.
Do not mistake "talk" for "action."
Pity fills no stomach.
Compassion builds no house.
Understanding is not yet justice.

—SHIMON BEN GAMLIEL[2]

God's holiest name is justice, and it is the just that keep the creation alive.

—KABBALAH

All authentic mystical traditions proclaim with one strong voice: the aim of awakening is not merely to realize one's own divine identity, but to serve all beings with humble joy and compassion and a commitment to justice on all levels and in all realms. The enlightened life is one that balances ecstatic inwardness with dedicated action, profound inner surrender with unceasing service to others. A great Indian saint, Anandamayi Ma, once said to a friend of Andrew Harvey's, "Just as God is both utterly peaceful and utterly dynamic, so the being who realizes God is at once sunk in a calm that nothing can disturb and active with a love that nothing can defeat. It is so simple;" she added, "through sacred practice you breathe in divine inspiration, divine strength, divine peace, and divine passion. Then you breathe them out in acts of wise compassion. This is the real life all of us are called to." The enlightened balance of the real that Anandamayi Ma describes has never been more precisely and majestically celebrated than in these words of the Upanishads:

In dark night live those for whom
The world without alone is real; in night
Darker still, for whom the world within
Alone is real. The first leads to a life
Of action, the second to a life of meditation.
But those who combine action with meditation
Cross the sea of death through action
And enter into immortality
Through the practice of meditation.
So have we heard from the wise.
In dark night live those for whom the Lord
Is transcendent only; in night darker still,
For who he is immanent only.
But those for whom he is transcendent
And immanent cross the sea of death
With the immanent and enter into
Immortality with the transcendent.
So have we heard from the wise.

—THE ISHA UPANISHADS[3]

Let all the great joys we have explored be lived and experienced in the depths of your body and in the full compassion of your spirit. Then your blissful sacred heart will awaken, longing to serve all beings everywhere in joy and boundless compassion. On his deathbed, Joseph Campbell turned to his wife, Jane, and grieved the way in which his remark "Follow your bliss" had been misused to justify narcissistic self-absorption. People had taken the phrase without putting it into the context of what he had actually said. Campbell's original quote was, "If you look for your bliss, you will find here is a place where your gift intersects where the hunger of the world exists."[4]

Grounded in an awakening luminous body, and rooted in the great peace of meditation, your sacred heart burns with the holy desire to see all beings safe, protected, and happy. This alchemical fire also longs to transform the ego-based illusions, institutions, and laws of the world so that they reflect the merciful all-embracing love of the Beloved.

Those who come to know and live in the sacred heart and act from its passion of compassion are Sacred Activists. Sacred Activists unite in their core the holy peace, strength, courage, and passion of the yoga of the Sacred Marriage with the holy desire of the heart to see justice established everywhere. They work whole-heartedly to see the poor housed and fed, the environment cherished and protected, and all sentient beings revered as divine, and so in turn experience the joy of the secret enshrined in these words of Chuang-Tzu:

> The more they give to themselves
> The more they can give to others:
> The more they give to others
> The more they have for themselves.[5]

It is the joy of this secret that gives the seeker the courage to pray, as the Dalai Lama prays in his practice every morning:

> May I be a guard for those who need protection
> A guide for those on the path
> A boat, a raft, a bridge for those who wish to cross the flood
> May I be a lamp in the darkness
> A resting place for the weary
> A healing medicine for all who are sick
> A vase of plenty, a tree of miracles
> And for the boundless multitudes of living beings
> May I bring sustenance and awakening
> Enduring like the earth and sky
> Until all beings are freed from sorrow
> And all are awakened.[6]

The true aim of Heart Yoga is not merely to help beings savor the great joys of the marriage, nor to facilitate the process of divinization of the body only. It is to birth, through the rigorous and devoted practice of the marriage of yoga and mysticism, devoted servants of a peaceful world community. This Great Turning, as Joanna Macy has called it,[7] is now taking place in the middle of, and partly as a result of, the global catastrophes that are threatening our planet. As the great Hopi prophecy states, "When earthquakes, floods, hailstorms, droughts, and famine will be the life of everyday, the time will then have come for the return to the true path."[8]

With bodies infused with the inspiration of the transcendent, and with mystical awareness grounded in the peace and stability of the immanent, those of us who have heeded the call to serve the creation of a new humanity will be able to devote ourselves whole-heartedly without growing exhausted. Through the ever-deepening experience of the power of the marriage of yoga and mysticism, we will find the strength and wisdom to serve all beings, and to live in deep peace and joy.

Through living and serving in this way, we will become the new humanity we long to establish. We will both embody the light and serve the light's compassionate desire to illuminate and awaken all beings.

The practice of yoga, when united with a precise and luminous mystical consciousness, offers an unshakeable foundation for the great work ahead. This is the great work we have been destined for since the beginning: the birthing of a humble, generous, tenderhearted, illumined divine humanity on Earth.

B. K. S. Iyengar, the great pioneer of the modern renaissance of yoga, writes in *Light on Life,* "It is no extravagant claim to say that wisdom has come to me by the practice of yoga, and the grace of God has lit the lamp in the inner core of me. This allows me to see the same light of the soul glowing in all other beings."[9]

From this wisdom, inspired by the vision that your illuminated inner core gives you, realize the ultimate purpose of embodying the light, which is to be a light for yourself and others, and to serve all beings with a full and glowing heart. As Iyengar guides us, "Be inspired but not proud. Do not aim low; you will miss the mark. Aim high, you will be on the threshold of bliss."[10]

Attune yourself to what serves you best, in this moment. To be of service in a sustainable way, you must know and respond to what you need. Choose whether you need a heating, awakening practice or a cooling, restorative practice to best prepare you for your karma yoga of the day.

When you sense that you need grounding or extra vitality, or if you're feeling distracted, unfocused, or not present, an active, heating practice can help you return to the strength of your body and restore your energy, intention, and clarity. Strengthening yoga postures develop courage and stamina for the practical healing, creative, and transformative work we do in the world, the karma yoga of Sacred Activism.

When you're not attending to the messages of your body or mind, it's easy to feel overwhelmed, ineffectual, stressed, or burned out. Reconnect directly with your own source of inspiration with a relaxing, restorative yoga practice. A restorative practice helps you to move beyond the boundaries of your ego to the place where the desire to serve others naturally arises. As B. K. S. Iyengar said, "Yoga releases the creative potential of life."[11] In this way the yoga practice of the Joy of Service truly serves all beings.

The Joy of Service Sequence: Energizing Yoga Practice

- Child's Pose – *Adho Mukha Virasana*
- Hands and Knees Pose
- Downward-facing Dog Pose – *Adho Mukha Svanasana*
- Sun Salutations – *Surya Namaskar*
  Part One, Drawing Down the Light
  Part Two, Sun Salutation Series
- Triangle Pose – *Trikonasana*
- Warrior Pose II – *Virbhadrasana II*
- Wide-legged Standing Forward Bend – *Prasarita Padottanasana*

- Warrior Pose I – *Virbhadrasana I*
- Standing Forward Bend – *Uttanasana*
- Sphinx Pose – *Bhujangasana* modification
- Cobra Pose – *Bhujangasana*
- Camel Pose – *Ustrasana*
- Bridge Pose – *Setu Bandhasana*
- Upward-facing Bow Pose – *Urdhva Dhanurasana*
- Bridge Pose – *Setu Bandhasana*
- Reclined Leg Release – *Supta Padangusthasana*
- Reclined Back Twist – *Jathara Parivartanasana* (modified)
- Back Releases
- Legs Up Wall Pose – *Viparita Karani*
- *Savasana*

Child's Pose
Adho Mukha Virasana
In the Child's Pose to celebrate the Joy of Service, you offer and surrender yourself—heart, mind, body, and soul—to the Beloved to be its instrument in the world.

Come to a kneeling position, slightly widening your knees. Sink your feet, shins, and thighs down into the earth while gently lifting your belly and heart. With an exhalation, slowly release your chest onto your thighs, resting your hands by your feet, palms soft like a baby's hands. Rest your forehead on your mat or on a bolster, curled into the position of the embryo.

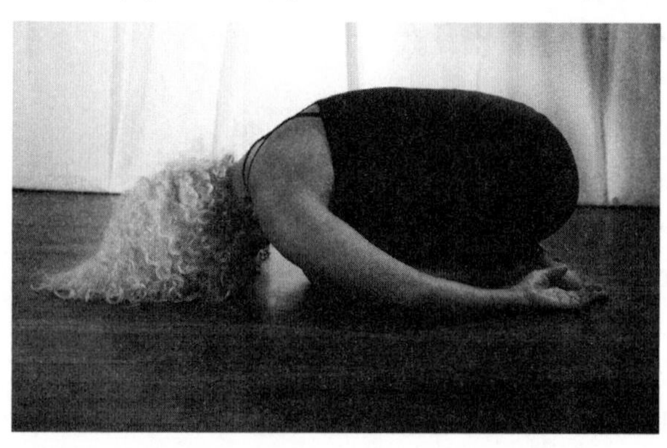

Relax in this position of prayer, melting into the strong loving arms of Mother Earth beneath you. Notice how your breath naturally flows into the backs of your lungs, which open your back ribs like feathers, and widen and release your kidneys. Let your back body open like spreading wings, lifting you into the spaciousness of Father Sky around and above you. With each breath, open every cell to the marriage of the Mother's warm energy rising from the earth with the blessing of the Father's infinite protection from above.

Imagine every cell breathing evenly. With profound devotion, pray that every cell can catch flame consciously in the fire of love. Imagine millions of soft fires igniting in your body-mind, and allow their glow to suffuse you entirely.

While keeping your focus on the light of the inner fires, slowly and tenderly lengthen your arms out in front of you. Bring your awareness to your breath, feeling it wash over you again and again, returning you to the root of your true self.

Commit yourself to serving all beings, inspired with the grace and peace that is suffusing you now. Remember to take this inspiration with you into all you do in the world.

Hands and Knees Pose

Slowly move to your hands and knees, feeling how they touch the earth. Gaze at your strong hands, looking at them as if you've never seen them before. Marvel at their intricacy and mystery, and all that they create in the world. See your fingers as rays radiating out from the suns at the center of your palms. Feel that strong, solar energy streaming up your hands, through your arms, into your heart, belly, and pelvis, and down your legs into your feet.

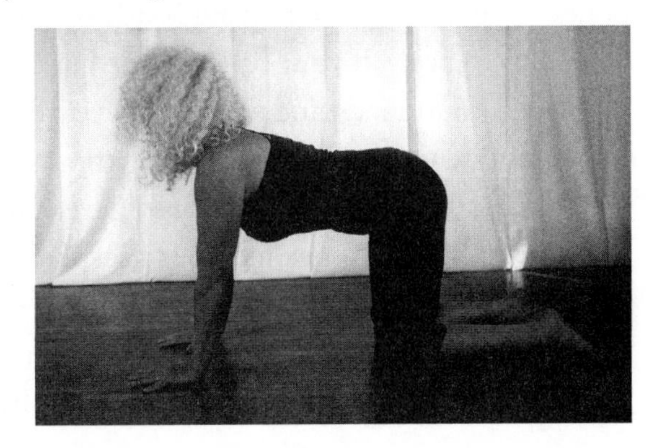

Inhale, lifting your tailbone and head, and dropping your belly. Feel your spine undulating through the core of your body like seaweed moving in a wave, releasing the front of your spine. As you exhale, draw your tailbone and head downward and arch your spine upward, the back of your spine now rippling open. Let your spine move back and forth with each breath.

Feel the spine's joyful release in the core of your body with the wave of each breath. Release into this rhythmic unity of body, heart, and breath.

Unravel your mind in the sensuous snake-like movement of your spine. Enjoy the sacred dance of your spine, hips, and shoulders. Become aware of the dynamic energy between your pubic bone and tailbone (See page 150 of the Joy of Tantra yoga practice sequence in Chapter Seven for a detailed description). Feel the vibration between these bones, and the powerful energy that flows up through the floor of your pelvis when the conscious connection between these bones is awakened. Draw this energy up into the core of your body, and bring this awareness of your core strength into the rest of your practice.

Downward-facing Dog Pose
Adho Mukha Svanasana

In Downward-facing Dog Pose, you will experience the stability of sending your roots down into the earth, while expanding in all directions into infinite space. In this pose, you humbly embody the marriage between transcendence and immanence, energizing your whole being.

From the hands and knees, curl your toes under. Imagine your belly is a helium balloon, lifting your hips up to the sky into Dog Pose. Elongate the bones of your spine like moving beads on a rosary, and lengthen your legs from hips to heels. If your back or legs hurt, keep your knees bent.

Embed your hands and feet into the earth, imagining them sinking into warm mud while your tailbone softly floats. Let your head drop, pouring all lingering thoughts like water onto the earth, quieting your mind. Feel the base of your skull loosen, and your neck soften. If you become tired, rest in Child's Pose, returning to Downward-facing Dog Pose when you feel ready.

Explore arching your back into a backbend like a dog bowing. Let it be a moving, flowing Dog Pose, paws stepping from side to side, tail wagging.

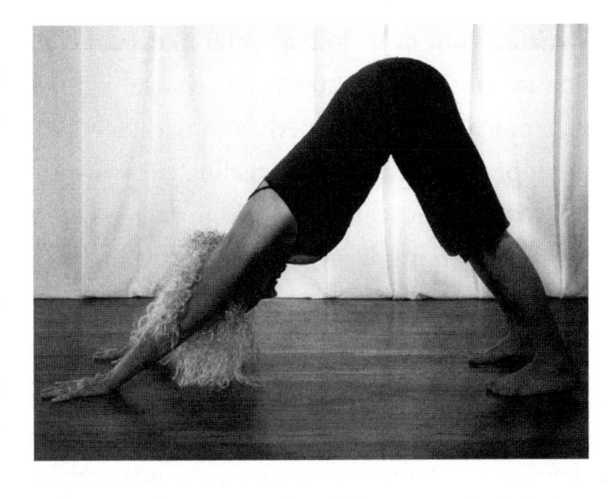

Swivel and spiral, and enjoy the playfulness and joy of being a dog. Listen to how your body wants to move. Step from foot to foot, bend your knees, or come up onto your toes. Let the joy and delight of exploration sparkle throughout every cell. (See page 69 for more details on this pose.)

Rest again in Child's Pose. Dedicate the energy that fills your whole being to the service of all beings.

> *My task ahead is like a rosary.*
> In the hours this work will take,
> Miracles will happen unobserved
> Within my body and mind.
> My spirit will grow in maturity.
> My love for humankind will make some new acquaintances.
> I will savor each second,
> Lay down each minute
> Carefully and joyously
> A brick in the temple of my being.
> *My task ahead is like a rosary.*
>
> —MODERN PRAYER FROM MADRID, SPAIN[12]

Sun Salutations
Surya Namaskar

Part One: Drawing Down the Light

Begin in *Tadasana* by surrounding yourself with a circle of golden light, and visualize your heart in the center like a softly pulsing sun. This image enables you to consciously enter your mystical light-body. When your visualization is strong and vivid, tenderly and with devotion draw your hands together in front of your heart center, feeling the warmth of your heart sun.

Uniting transcendence and immanence, the Sun Salutation invokes the all-transforming light-energy of the sun. This Shakti energy awakens our subtle energy centers and illuminates every cell. By practicing Sun Salutation as a profound prayer, we unveil the embodied suns that we are and experience the holy joy of living as the Light.

We breathe in the solar energy and breathe it out as an offering back to the Source. We invoke it as the foundation for our service to all beings and become embodied suns, worshipping our Mother-Father, the great Sun. When we practice with this consciousness, gratitude and bliss suffuse our whole being, and the power of transcendent energy ignites every cell, strengthening us for our work in the world.

Pressing the roots of your thumbs into your heart center, feel your heart pulsing with light-energy. Bow your head slightly so that your head rests in the soft, warm, luminous bed of your heart.

Open your hands and release your arms down to your sides, palms turned out. Feel your arms and hands extend from the core of your heart. Become aware of the vibrant line of energy streaming from the heart sun, through your shoulders and down your arms into the glow of your fingertips.

Let your arms slowly rise like wings spreading from your heart center. Experience the light radiating from you, and with your hands draw that circle of golden light around you. As your hands gradually come together, feel the connection of your left and right sides joining as one. Sense how your fingertips flare upwards from the sun of your heart, your belly, and your feet.

Empowered by the light-energy you have invoked, now gratefully draw down that divine radiance into the core of your body, awakening your sacred centers.

Very slowly lowering your joined palms, pull the transcendent light down through the crown of your head. As you do so, visualize the crown chakra opening like a thousand-petaled lotus of diamond light.

Continue slowly drawing down the light through your third eye, awakening and visualizing it as a diamond eye streaming light in all directions.

Continuing down through the center in your throat, visualize that center opening as a rich red rose, illumined from within by soft golden light.

Bring your hands to rest in front of your heart, visualizing your heart center as a burning golden chalice, glowing with light. This glowing chalice within you is the sacred heart. It holds the fountain of strength that will give you the courage, inspiration, and stamina to go on offering service to others. In this position of profound empowerment and prayer, let the sacred heart within you speak these words of St. Francis:

> Lord, make me an instrument of thy peace.
> Where there is hatred, let me sow love;
> Where there is injury, pardon;
> Where there is doubt, faith;
> Where there is despair, hope;
> Where there is darkness, light;
> Where there is sadness, joy.
> O divine Master, grant that I may not so much seek
> To be consoled as to console,
> To be understood as to understand,
> To be loved as to love;
> For it is in giving that we receive;
> It is in pardoning that we are pardoned;
> It is in dying that we are born to eternal life.
>
> —FRANCIS OF ASSISI[13]

Feel the simplicity of simply standing on planet Earth, with your feet rooted on the earth below and the crown of your head open to the light above. The sacred energies of earth and heaven meet and merge in the marriage bed of your heart.

Sun Salutation
Surya Namaskar

Part Two: Sun Salutation Series

From *Tadasana,* open and empty your hands and sweep your arms out, letting the golden wings of your heart open. Join your hands above you and then open them out to the sides, sweeping your arms down from your heart as you bow forward. Hinge deeply from the hip joints, bending your knees if that is more comfortable for you. Release your hands to the earth, and touch it with reverence. Slowly slide one foot back, and then the other, balancing in the Plank Pose (like a high push-up position).

From Plank Pose, you can either: release your knees, chest, and chin to the floor then lift your heart up, like the sun rising, into a simple Cobra Pose (See page 106); or if you have the strength, release down into a low push-up position then straighten your arms, lifting your heart up.

From Cobra or Upward-facing Dog Pose, either rest in Child's Pose or go directly into Downward-facing Dog Pose.

From Dog Pose, bend your knees and lengthen back into the total surrender of Child's Pose. Release your forehead onto the floor, softening your eyes, quieting your mind, and resting on the earth.

Feel the blessing of your body kissing the earth, and let this blessing inspire you to offer your life gratefully in loving service to all beings.

Now slowly sweep forward again to your hands and knees. Curl your toes under, lift your belly, and come back to Downward-facing Dog Pose. Step one foot forward between your hands, again coming into a lunge, and then bring the other foot forward, returning to the Forward Bend. Bend your knees, rise up through your belly and heart, and sweep your arms out to the sides and over your head as you float up to standing.

Again draw the light down with your palms joined, through the thousand-petaled lotus of the crown chakra, through the diamond light of the third eye, through the rich red rose of the throat, into the luminous golden chalice of the heart. Arrive back in the sacred heart center, with gratitude and wonder.

Return to Mountain Pose *(Tadasana)*, lifting your heart, your eyes softly gazing into the light. Your feet are firmly on earth, while your sacred heart opens both to the transcendent and, in great compassion, to all sentient beings. Commit yourself to being a humble midwife to the great birth, offering yourself body, mind, and heart in service. Repeat the Sun Salutation three times, allowing your breath to lead you. Remember throughout that this practice is one of the holiest of prayers.

Triangle Pose
Trikonasana

In the Triangle Pose for the Joy of Service, you can experience the mystery of your embodiment as a human being. You are the vibrating link between heaven and earth, and the conduit and servant of divine energy on Earth.

Step your feet a wide distance apart (one meter or more), anchoring them into the earth. Turn your left foot in slightly, and your right foot out 90 degrees, keeping your body facing forward. Spread your arms wide, at shoulder height, palms down. Elongate from the front of your heart into your middle fingers, and from the back of your heart into your little fingers. In Chinese medicine this gesture opens the heart and pericardium meridians, thereby releasing a healing flow of energy that floods the whole bodymind.

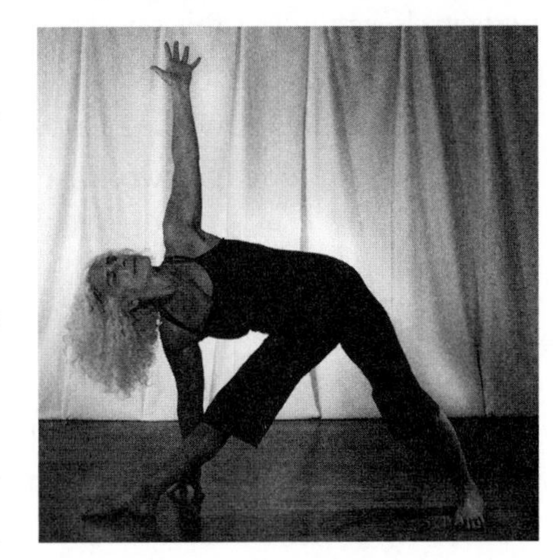

Rest your arms on this flowing line of energy as if they were floating on clouds. Listen to the dancing dialog between your tailbone and the crown of your head, as spaces open between the bones of your spine. Experience your rootedness on earth as well as your soaring connection with sky. Feel your vital energy radiating evenly from your core like a starfish through the five directions of the legs, arms, and head.

Inhale, lifting the sides of your waist, then exhale and lengthen over to the right side, placing your right hand on a block or your leg for support, while lifting up through the left arm. Balance evenly through your arms and legs as you elongate from your tailbone to the crown of your head.

Feel a sensation of ease and steadiness flowing throughout your body. Stay here for a few breaths, experiencing your body as an open channel between earth and heaven, firmly rooted on earth while opening like a light-flower into heaven. Let your breath lead you as you come up and repeat this pose to the other side.

In Triangle Pose you celebrate and express the mystery of being the intersection between absolute and relative, heaven and earth, the divine child born from the marriage of the transcendent father and the embodied mother. Triangle Pose embodies in a simple and directly accessible way this triune mystery, the mystery of the three: the father, mother, and child; the transcendent, immanent, and creation; or in the Christian formulation, the Father, Son, and Holy Spirit, in which the Holy Spirit is the mother force of love. In this pose the body itself symbolizes this mystery by creating a variety of triangles.

Whenever you are ready, come up from Triangle Pose and return to Mountain Pose. Dedicate the energy that Triangle Pose gives you to the work that you wish to do in the world.

Warrior Pose II
Virbhadrasana II

In Warrior Pose II for the Joy of Service practice you embody the strength and courage you need to do your true work in the world.

Spread your feet about four feet apart, grounding them in the earth beneath

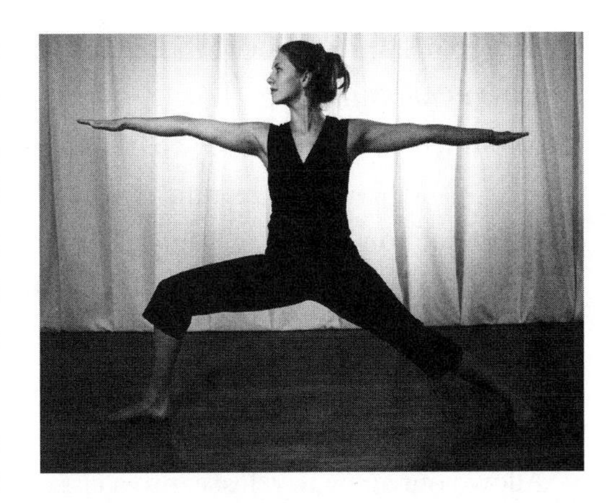

you. Feel the strength in your legs; they are the warrior's foundation. Rooted in Mother Earth, the warrior receives stability and stamina. Turn your right foot out 90 degrees and your left foot in 45 degrees. Spread your arms out to the sides at shoulder height.

Slowly release your right hip, bringing your right knee over your right ankle, while maintaining the rootedness of your left leg. Your right leg forms a right angle. To protect your knee be sure that it is externally rotating so that it points to the little-toe side of your right foot. Balance evenly over the midline of your body, perfectly poised in this moment, neither clinging to the past nor lunging forward into the future. Turn your head back to look at your left hand and awaken it, then turn your head again to gaze beyond your right hand. Take a few breaths here, and then come up and practice Warrior Pose II to the other side.

Lift between your tailbone and pubic bone to support the opening of your heart. Feel the beauty and the dignity of this position. Imagine that you're a spiritual warrior, poised at the edge of a cliff, looking down at the battlefield of life below. Gaze out over all creation, while still feeling your feet firmly rooted on this earth.

Stabilize yourself in Warrior Pose, finding your roots and standing firmly in all that you are in this moment, balanced between your past and your future. Your legs strongly connect with the earth, energy rising up through the marriage bed of the pelvic floor into your heart, and into the spacious canopy of your mind.

Return to *Tadasana* when you are ready. Let your whole body-mind be grounded in the dignity and courage of the spiritual warrior, who is willing to give everything for love.

Wide-legged Standing Forward Bend
Prasarita Padottanasana
Step your feet a wide distance apart and turn them parallel. Take your hands to the tops of your thighs and slowly move your thighs back, feeling the earthiness of your legs. Let your pelvis release forward over the tops of your thighbones, elongating your spine and shining your heart energy forward. You can put your fingertips onto a block, or place your hands on the floor beneath your shoulders. If you feel any strain in your back or knees, bend your knees or come up.

Allow your spine to release into a crescent moon shape, blending the lunar, receptive energy of your spine with the solar, dynamic energy of your legs.

Enjoy the steadiness of your legs supporting the surrender of your spine; the marriage within your body of strength and softness. Your lower body is firmly grounded while your upper body flows over like a waterfall.

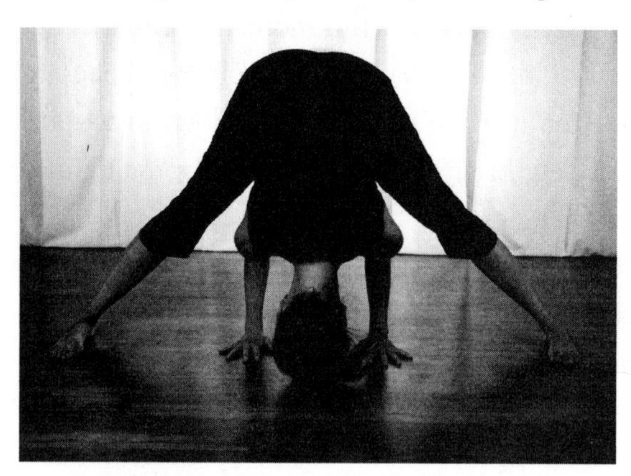

Let these powerful words from the classic yogic text, the Bhagavad Gita, inspire you with the courage to assume the work in the world for which you are destined.

> If you say, "I will not fight this battle,"
> Your own nature will drive you into it.
> If you will not fight the battle of life,
> Your own karma will drive you into it.
> The Lord dwells in the hearts of all creatures,
> And he whirls them round on the wheel of time.
> Run to him for refuge with all your strength
> And peace profound will be yours through his grace.[14]

Keeping your legs steady, inhale and come up when you are ready, returning to *Tadasana.* (See page 39 for more details on this pose.)

Warrior Pose I
Virbhadrasana I

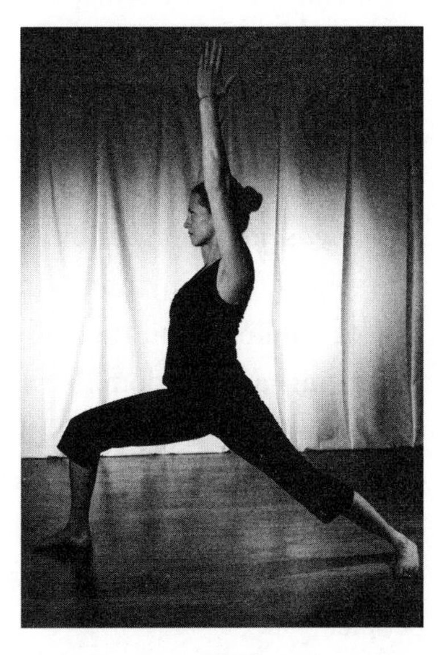

Step your feet about four feet apart. Turn your left foot in at a 45-degree angle, and your right foot out 90 degrees. Rotate your hips to face the short end of your mat, keeping your back foot rooted into the earth. Press down through your right foot, and release your right leg into a right angle. From your heart, sweep your arms over your head, palms facing each other. Stay for three to five breaths, lifting through your pelvic floor, scooping the belly toward the back of the diaphragm. Come up and repeat the pose on the other side. Breathe in the strong warrior energy surging into your spiritual warrior's sacred heart, and with your exhalation, offer this energy out in service to all beings. Return to *Tadasana.*

Standing Forward Bend
Uttanasana

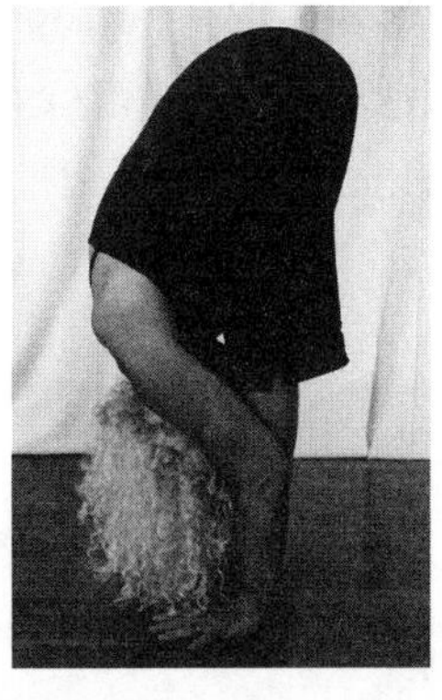

From *Tadasana,* bring your hands to the tops of your thighbones and gently slide them back behind you, aligning your hips, knees, and ankles. Lifting your sitting bones, tip your pelvis forward over the tops of your thighs and let your spine evenly round forward into a rainbow arc. You may bend your knees slightly to protect your back.

Make a cradle of your arms, and rest your hands on the opposite elbows, or rest your hands on a block, on your legs, or on the floor. Release your head, softening your neck. Relax for a few breaths, surrendering into this pose. Feel the strength and earthiness of your legs, the fluidity of your pelvis, the warmth in your heart, and the joy of being present in your re-energized spiritual warrior's body. Bend your knees and come into Child's Pose, then slide forward onto your belly and release your front body onto the earth.

Sphinx Pose
***Bhujangasana* modification**
The sphinx of the pyramids in ancient Egypt is a mythical creature with the face of a human and the body of a lion. This archetypal symbol expresses the serenity and wisdom that are attained when the human being unveils and enters into her identity with all creation. From experiencing this identity with creation in the pose of the sphinx, your natural inclination to serve others is renewed, and you begin to understand the mystery that many teachers reveal when they say that you never serve *other* people because there are no *other* people.

In Sphinx Pose, you are invited to savor and claim the full power of this enigmatic symbol, tasting the wonder of your own deepest secrets. Let the pose of the sphinx speak to you as it spoke to the Pharaohs, Oedipus, and to Alexander the Great, revealing the magical depth of your identity with all that exists.

Keeping your belly soft, curl your spine up slightly and slide your elbows underneath your shoulders. Pressing the palms of your hands down into the earth, widen and lift your collarbones. Roll from leg to leg, drawing your inner legs toward each other until the two begin to feel like one leg, grounded in the earth. Slowly and majestically lift your head, smiling serenely. Lift your belly softly toward your heart.

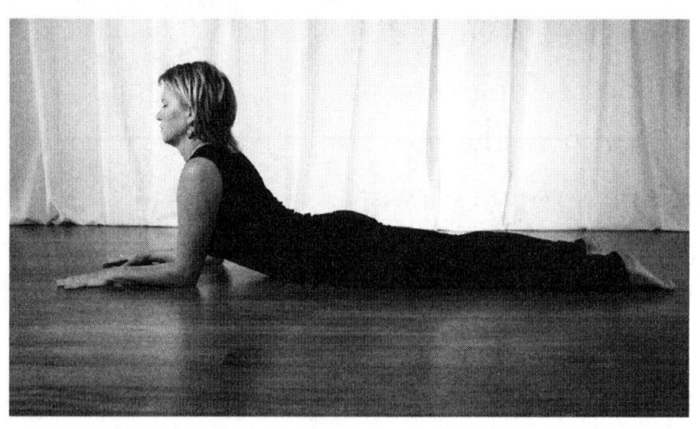

You will feel the warm energy flowing from your lion heart into your head and flooding your human consciousness. Like the sphinx, radiate the lion's compassion and courage to all creatures. Human and animal spiral into each other along the gentle curling current of the spine.

Slowly release down to the floor, unraveling all the cells of your body. Feel them glow with the serene energy of the heart's nectar. When you are ready, slowly rise up again, repeating Sphinx Pose a few times.

Let the realization of your human/animal connection with all creation awaken your heart center.

Cobra Pose
Bhujangasana

Soften your belly onto the earth like a golden king cobra. Elongate your spine, and feel it undulating and spiraling throughout its length. Rest here and release your body, with the king cobra's regal confidence, into the dark, rich warmth of the earth below.

In Cobra Pose, you will experience and incarnate the ancient power and sacred wisdom that has in many cultures been associated with the snake. A creature at ease both in the dark worlds of the earth and in the worlds of light, the snake effortlessly fuses the energy and knowledge of both. It is a perfect guide for the Sacred Activist, for in his or her own being are married spiritual awareness and passion to serve all beings.

In the classical yoga system, the divine energy referred to as "kundalini" is said to be coiled at the base of the spine and is depicted as a coiled snake. When this energy is uncoiled, it shoots its fiery power up through all the sacred centers to explode into what is described as a thousand-petaled lotus of light in the crown center. This

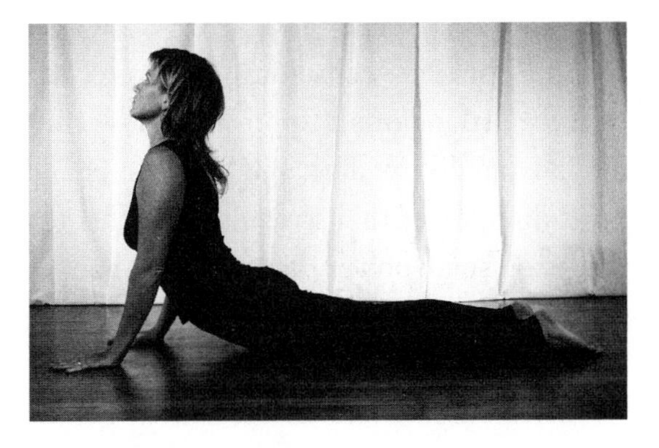

explosion could be conceived as the divine orgasm of the union between father and mother, transcendence and immanence, and it births the yogi into the bliss energy and knowledge of divine consciousness.

In Hinduism, the god of yogis, Shiva, is often represented with a cobra curled around his right upper arm. This symbolizes the union of spacious sky consciousness with primordial earth energy into which the practice of yoga initiates its devotees.

Slide your hands under your shoulders, and press them down into the earth. Experience the strength of your legs that flows into your pelvis from the arches of your feet. Allow the front of your hips and legs to lengthen, rolling your legs slightly inward. Invite your tailbone toward your pubic bone.

Gently begin to coil your spine by lifting your belly toward the back of your heart, and let your shoulder blades begin to move forward, widening your collarbones. Lift your chest, your spine evenly coiling, without feeling any strain in your low back. Feel the strength of your arms and legs, and the sensuous power of the cobra. From the movement of your royal cobra heart, slowly lift your head. After a few breaths, slowly roll down, softening your belly back to earth. Repeat Cobra Pose a few times.

Feel the snake's smoothness of sensation spreading evenly through your body. In Sanskrit, this evenness of sensation is referred to as *sama,* the root word of "Samadhi." Samadhi is the highest expression of this sameness as absolute consciousness, a consciousness that experiences the One Taste of everything.

Let Cobra Pose consciously awaken you to your own inmost knowledge of the marriage of all opposites, masculine and feminine, earth and sky, human and divine, dark and light, body and spirit, and to the ever-flowing kundalini power that streams from this marriage when it is realized. It is this astonishing power that will give the Sacred Activist the endless supplies of loving energy that s/he will need to meet the demands of work in the world.

After your last Cobra Pose, slowly roll down, softening your snake belly back to earth. Rest for a few breaths, then elongate and release your spine in a gentle Dog Pose. Bring your knees to the floor, and sit in Hero Pose (See page 78).

Camel Pose

Ustrasana

Sitting back on your heels, press down through your feet and legs. Lift your sitting bones up away from your heels. Anchor your pelvis by dropping your tailbone toward the earth. Curl your toes under and open the arches of your feet. Bring your hands prayerfully to your heart. With your inhalation lift your heart; with your exhalation, curl your tailbone slightly forward and elongate your spine.

Stream energy down into the earth from your hips to your knees. Your belly lifts up into your heart center, and your collarbones rise and spread wide. Reach your fingertips back and place them on your heels. If that is too far to reach, place your hands on blocks, leave your hands on your heart, or place them on the backs of your legs.

Stay in this heart-releasing position of love and joy for a few breaths, and then slowly return your sitting bones to your heels, drawing your tailbone toward the floor to lengthen your lower back. Keep your heart lifted, radiating the golden light of compassion in all directions. Repeat Camel Pose several times, returning to Hero Pose to rest.

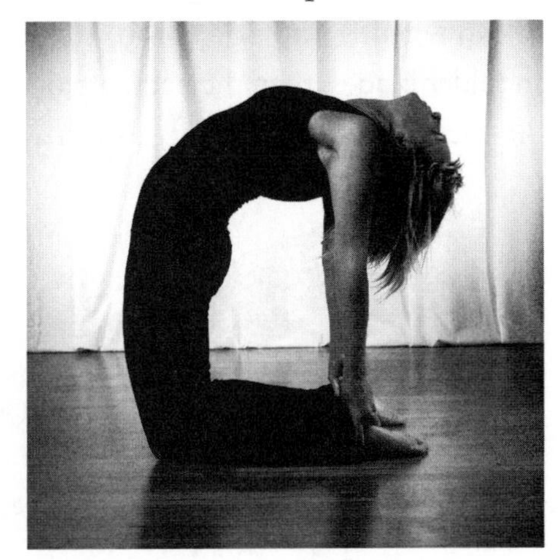

Without compressing your lower back, keep lifting your heart and feel it expanding and spreading in luminous space.

Open the chalice of your heart so that the divine honey can pour in, and drink the honey of your heart. Send the joy of this pose out to all beings as an offering of your love.

> Now may every living thing, young or old,
> Weak or strong, living near or far, known or unknown, living or departed or yet unborn,
> may every living thing be full of bliss.
>
> —THE BUDDHA[15]

From your heart radiate the warmth of your intention to serve all beings.

Bridge Pose

Setu Bandhasana

Roll onto your back, bending your knees and placing your feet parallel to each other, hip width apart. Press them down, embedding them into the floor. Notice the earthiness of your feet and the strength of your legs. Feel this Mother Earth energy lovingly infuse the minutest channels of your leg bones, and follow its warm flow up into your pelvis.

Lift your tailbone slightly up off the floor, curling it toward your pubic bone. Let this movement initiate the lift of your sitting bones off the floor. A flow of energy, originating from the arches of your feet, enters the sacred space between your tailbone and your pubic bone. This energy lifts your belly and hips up from the floor, your belly floating toward the sky, and your heart rising.

Now gently roll down onto the floor, first coming down between your shoulder blades, then the back of your waist, and then your tailbone, uncurling each vertebra mindfully as if it were a precious string of pearls. Notice how your front body begins to soften into the embrace of your broad back body. Repeat Bridge Pose a few times.

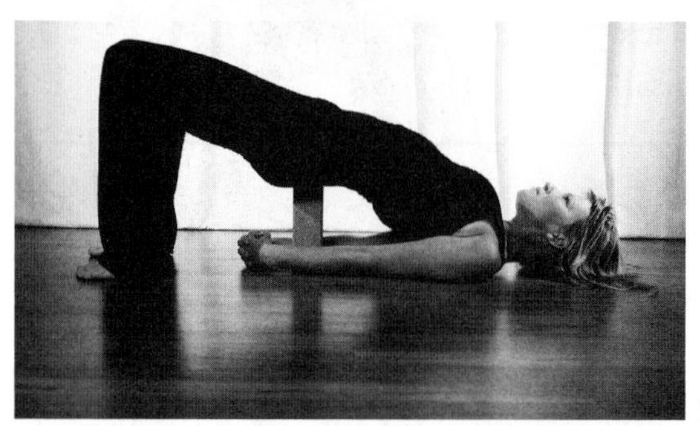

Let your heart energy brim over into your head and your mind flood with its tender, loving warmth. As this heart energy flows into your arms, press them strongly down into the earth. The strength of your arms and legs supports your spine in a rainbow arc, while your belly and heart float softly on this luminous arc. Allow your spine to relax into a gently rounded crescent moon.

In this pose you experience the body celebrating its inherent nature as a bridge between earth and sky. Slowly return back to earth, and dedicate this calm, steady energy to the work you do in the world.

Upward-facing Bow Pose
Urdvha Dhanurasana

(Do not practice this pose with back or wrist injury, during the last six months of pregnancy, or during the menstrual flow.)

In this ecstatic pose, the absolutely open heart is supported by the strength and calm of the absolutely balanced body. It symbolizes the necessity of a strong, unwavering connection with the earth beneath you as the foundation from which you whole-heartedly offer yourself in service.

To give to others in a healthy way, you need to be grounded in yourself. Similarly in this pose, to open your heart and offer yourself in love you first sink your roots down deep into your feet and into the earth. From that grounded security, firmly centered in the immanent, you can fully open yourself in love to the transcendent.

The asana is itself the manifestation of the marriage. It gives us a sublime and practical key to entering the fullness of the marriage. Establish yourself in the depths of your body as you simultaneously open your whole heart, mind, and being to Love. A tree cannot grow into its full majesty unless its roots are entwined deep into the earth.

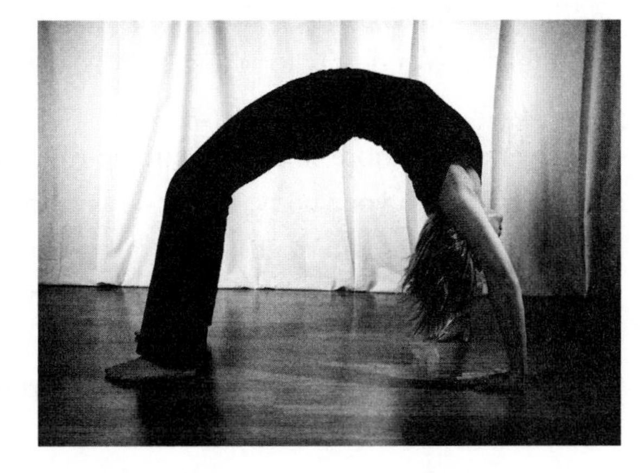

Doing the pose with this awareness will awaken you to the vibrant balance called for by a life of service. When you open yourself to the infinite wellspring of love energy that is always flowing within you, serving others comes naturally and is sustainable.

Explore this pose as an offering from the core of your heart and body, rather than trying to push into it as a test of your will or endurance. As Iyengar writes, "When you do the asana correctly the Self opens by itself; this is divine yoga."[16]

Experiment carefully with this intense backbend. Lying on your back, bend your knees and place your feet parallel and hip width apart near your sitting bones. Bring your hands underneath your shoulders, fingers pointing back toward your heels and turned a bit to the outside. Your hands can be placed slightly wider than your shoulders, so that your elbows will stay over your hands when you rise up.

Rock your pelvis, moving your tailbone toward your pubic bone, and your pubic bone toward your tailbone. Exhale and curl your tailbone up. Let this subtle movement initiate the rising of your hips off the floor. Move down into the earth through your hands and arms, and draw your shoulder blades into your body, lifting your chest. You may wish to first rest the crown of your head lightly on the floor, being careful that you don't compress your neck.

Engage your shoulder blades into the back ribs, and your arm bones firmly into your shoulder sockets. Make sure your feet and legs are parallel and hip width apart. Strongly press down through your hands and feet, and unroll into a full backbend. Stay for a few breaths, then slowly and mindfully release down to the floor.

Repeat a few more times, practicing rolling your spine up rather than forcing it up into your body. Move down through your legs, and open the fronts of your hips and thighs. Lift your tailbone up, releasing your sacrum deeply into your body and elongating through your lower back. Allow your spine to curl into an even roundedness, supported by the strength of your arms and legs. Keep your belly soft, your heart lifting, and your breath easy and flowing.

Come down to the floor whenever you feel ready, resting and then repeating the pose several times. When you release down to earth, rest and radiate out the intense energy that has flooded you to all sentient beings. This energy comes both from the strong support of the earth and from the transcendent shining its light down upon you. The impassioned strength of this pose fills every cell of your body with the renewed energy you can now offer in your ongoing service in the world.

Bridge Pose
Setu Bandhasana

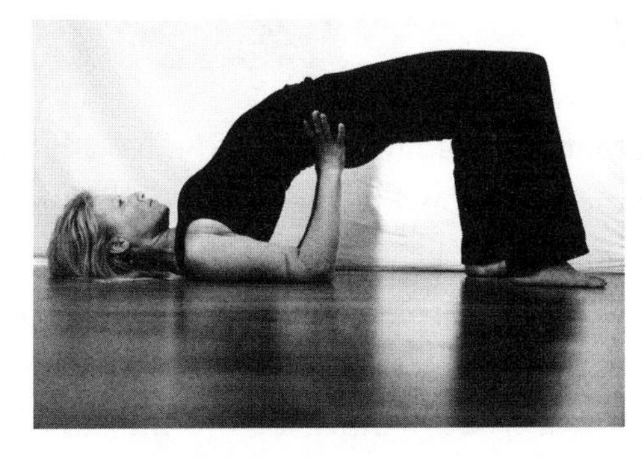

After Upward-facing Bow Pose, explore another gentle Bridge Pose to release your spine. Experiment with lengthening your fingers down toward your heels, turning your palms up, clasping your hands, or placing your hands under your hips. Practice without any pushing or struggle, coming up with ease and staying only as long as feels right.

When you come back down to the floor after Bridge Pose, do a few more gentle pelvic tilts, releasing and relaxing your back and belly. Allow your belly to stay quiet, like a still pool deep in the middle of the forest. Sense the warm glowing fire of your heart. Feel the joy of letting your body open so freely, and of opening your heart so naturally to love and service.

Reclined Leg Release
Supta Padangusthasana

Hug your right knee gently to your chest. Notice how the right side of your back opens and releases, and your internal organs on the right side soften. Slowly lengthen your left leg, moving out through your left heel and awakening your left foot.

Allow energy to spread throughout your entire body into every cell. Hold your right leg or place a strap around your right foot and slowly straighten

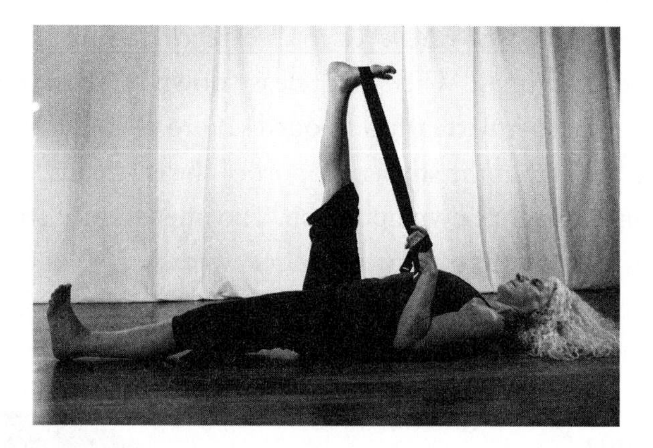

that leg, holding the strap with both hands and resting your shoulders on the floor. Stay fully present throughout your whole body in this pose, rather than just concentrating on your leg.

Keep your left leg dropping down toward the floor, elongating through your left heel, and releasing your low back. Your left leg rolls slightly to the inside, your right leg a bit to the outside, to maintain an even alignment of your pelvis.

After at least five breaths, fold your right knee back to your chest and then place the sole of your right foot on the floor. Slowly draw the heel of this foot down your mat, lengthening and releasing your right leg. Rest a few breaths before repeating this pose on the other side.

Reclined Back Twist

Lying on your back, exhale and draw your right knee up toward your chest. Move slowly and consciously, feeling your back opening and releasing to the earth. Relax the skin on your face and release your lower jaw. With each inhalation, soften your eyes. Lengthen your left leg onto the floor, elongating through your left heel. Strongly awaken your left foot, as if it were standing on the wall across from you. Spread your heart energy all the way down into both feet.

Now slowly roll your right knee across your body toward your left side, resting it on a folded blanket or block. Gently place your left hand on your

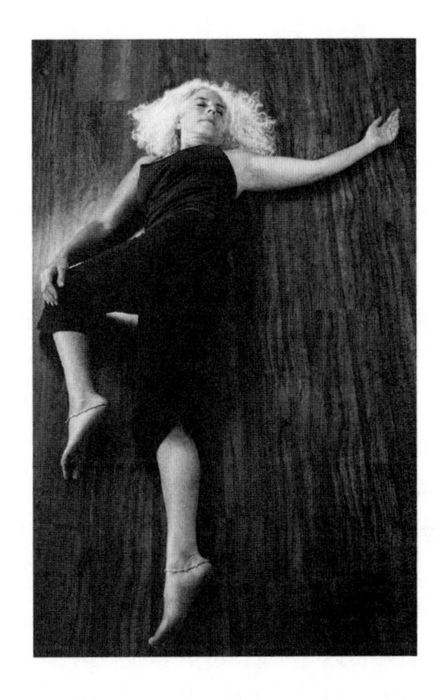

right knee. Take your right hand to your lower back. With the exhalation, feel how your tailbone slightly lengthens and delicately moves toward your pubic bone. With your inhalation, the pubic bone moves toward your tailbone. Notice the subtle dancing energy between your pubic bone and your tailbone.

From your pelvic floor, draw your awareness up toward your heart. Inhaling, fill your chest, and exhaling, release your right arm behind you. Notice how the area around your heart feels as you move your arm. Your belly lifts up toward your heart, and your heart energy radiates and streams out your arm.

If you feel any tension or tenderness in your back, modify this position so that it feels easier and more comfortable. You can take your right hand to your back and massage it. Bring a healing touch to wherever your body needs it, and notice how soothing the touch of your hand can be on your own body.

Imagine a golden light entering your open heart. Your heart is like a glowing chalice receiving the divine golden honey pouring into it.

Feel how the inhalation widens the area around your heart, and the exhalation deeply softens your heart space. Draw your body and breath together with the gentle focus of your mind.

In the Reclined Back Twist, your heart blossoms open like a flower of light radiating love energy throughout the channel of your arm and out through your fingertips behind you into the world. In this heart-releasing and heart-expanding position, imagine that you are receiving a downpouring of compassionate light from the Beloved, like a golden rain upon your body. Radiate it outward to all beings. Pray that this golden love energy, the energy of the sacred heart, can descend as peace on all sentient beings.

When you are ready to move, slowly come back to the center, drawing both knees up to your chest. As your back body widens and releases, rock gently back and forth. Rest here a few breaths before exploring the twist to the other side.

In the Reclined Back Twist, the intense and ecstatic offering of the heart in the Camel and Upward-facing Bow poses is experienced at a gentler depth. The passionate and fiery energy of those poses is distilled into a tender experience of love and union with all things. Through this pose, the passionate fire of divine love at its most exposed is alchemized into a quiet and blissful tenderness that is the foundation for a ceaseless flow of love-energy.

St. John of the Cross describes the transformation of the heart in the fire of love as having three stages. First, the log of the ordinary self, covered with the moss and lichens of confusion, is placed in the fire and starts to spit and crackle as it is purified. Then, as the fire of love enters the log more and more completely, it flares up in exuberant flame. Lastly, in the third stage, the flames of passion transform into the embers of an infinitely soft and tender glow that, as St. John says, "helps us enter the tenderness of the life of God."[17]

When it feels like the same amount of time on the second side, slowly return to the center, hugging both knees to your chest.

Once you have experienced, through grace and by your practice of yoga, the realization of this holy and tender absorption into love, you discover that it is from this soft fire that the calm strength and energy flows to radiate love outward to all beings. The paradox revealing itself here is that by reaching the most intimate union within ourselves, we find the source of a deathless power to love and continue serving others in boundless compassion. Inspired by this revelation and sustained by its power, there is nothing we cannot face and no task too grueling to undertake with patience, energy, and surrender.

Back Releases

These positions offer many options to explore letting go and resting. Lie on your back and hug your knees toward you. Rock from side to side, or from top to bottom, massaging your back on the floor. Cross your legs with one shin on top of the other as if sitting cross-legged, and release your knees toward the floor. Cross your legs with the other shin on top, and bring awareness to your breath.

Visualize your heart flowering open with your inhalation, and your belly releasing and relaxing with your exhalation, each breath gently cradling the heart. Rest your knees on each other, your feet flat on the floor, or take the soles of your feet together. Allow your back to melt into the earth.

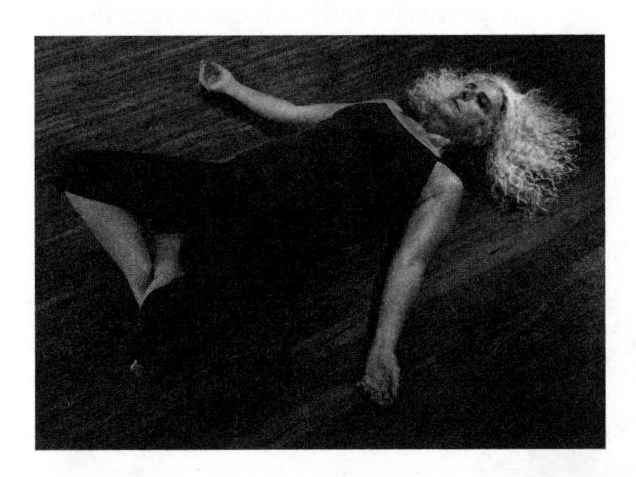

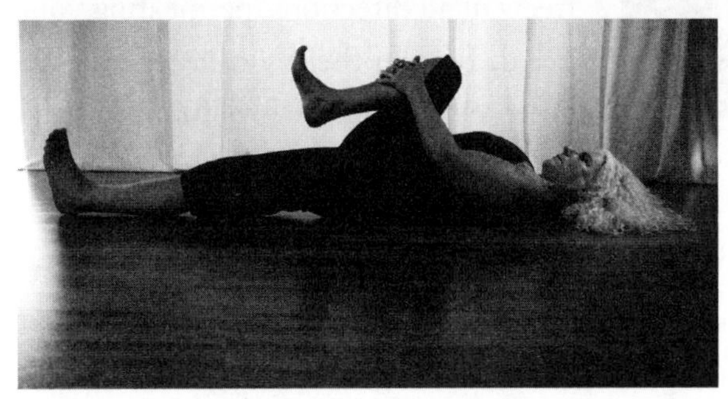

Legs Up Wall Pose
Viparita Karani
Sit with one hip close to a wall, then swing around and put your legs up the wall. Your back can rest on the floor, or you can place a support under your hips and chest to elevate your torso slightly while your shoulders rest on the floor. This creates a gentle roundedness throughout your chest. If it feels like your chin is lifting too much, place a small pillow under your head and neck to support the curve of your neck, and adjust your forehead so that it's higher than your chin.

Spread your arms to the sides, opening your heart center, and turn your palms up. Release the tops of your thighbones toward the wall, softening your belly with each exhalation. If your legs or back feel uncomfortable, adjust the distance of your hips from the wall, or bend your legs slightly. An eye pillow softens the gaze inward.

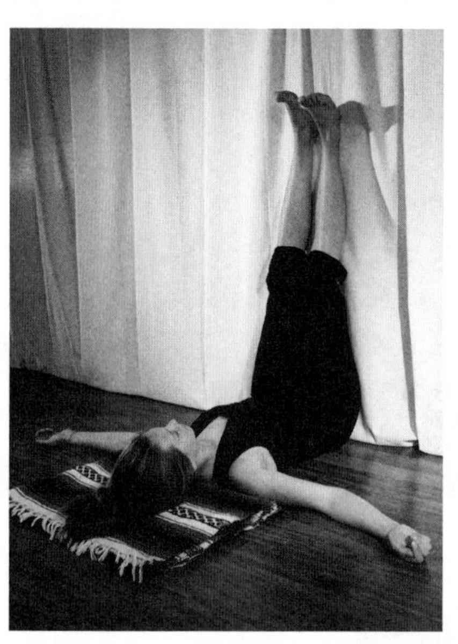

Observe how tension and tiredness drain down your legs, and energy flows like a waterfall into the quiet pool of your pelvis, brimming back into your heart and head. The breath releases your chest, and heart energy flows freely in all directions, permeating your mind. Rest in the joy of release, your heart awake in pure love for all beings.

Savasana
In this *Savasana* for the Joy of Service, we offer our entire body, mind, heart, and soul on the altar of love. We ask love to so suffuse our every cell that we become love's instrument of service to all beings.

Sit on your mat with your knees up and your feet flat. Release back to your elbows, and pause to let your belly drop back. Feel your kidneys release, and the back of your waist lengthen. Elongate your back as you relax onto the floor. Place an eye pillow over your eyes. Extend your arms down to the sides, turning your palms up so that the hands are soft, just like babies' hands. Feel your back body widening, and your front body releasing back.

Simply notice the natural inclination of your body to melt back into the earth, your body flowing down like water running downhill. Release back into the cauldron of the earth beneath you. Feel the comfort of being able to lie back and let go, like a child snuggling back into its mother's arms. The boundaries of your body soften and become amorphous, like a cloud dissolving in the sky.

When thoughts arise, let them float in the spacious blue sky of your mind. Feel the breath gently flowing through your body like a wave washing through you. As you notice your body beginning to relax and settling back into the silence, observe your mind also gradually beginning to settle. Experience the truth of Patanjali's explanation of yoga (Yoga Sutras, I-2) as the dissolving of the thought waves of the mind back into their source.

Your skin becomes more porous and transparent, almost translucent, so that the light of your innermost self radiates from you in all directions, and the light surrounding you permeates your body from all sides, turning you into a brilliant diamond, a crystallization of the divine light surrounding you.

Visualize bathing yourself in waves of this light. Consciously breathe this diamond light in and out. See the diamond light constantly descending in blessing, and offer yourself to it in prayer and gratitude. With each inhalation, absorb the light more and more deeply, and with each exhalation, effortlessly radiate it out, dedicating it to the service and liberation of all beings. Rest in *Savasana* as long as you wish.

From the spaciousness of *Savasana*, gently draw your awareness to your breath. With the body so relaxed and receptive, notice how freely the breath flows. The doors and the windows of the body are open, so that the exquisite cooling and cleansing light-winds of the breath can wash through and renew you.

Allow these winds of breath to awaken your body-mind, bathing each cell in this dawn light of renewal. Feel the extremely subtle transformation on the minutest molecular level that this immersion in the light-energy awakens in your body.

Gradually let the breath bring you fully present into this moment. Feel your body resting on the earth, its shape, and the vital energy pulsing through it.

When you feel ready, move from the position of the corpse, *Savasana,* rolling onto your right side into the position of the embryo, of birth, feeling the support of the whole earth beneath you as you turn. Feel that you are being birthed in every cell of your body as a divine/human being, the divine child. Rest on your mother, Mother Earth, the way a baby rests on its mother's body. Feel the tenderness of her support, and the surrender of your being to her, so that she can awaken you to ever greater and more luminous depths of yourself.

At your own rhythm, when you feel like moving, slowly support yourself up to a sitting position. Sit as the divine golden radiant human being that you are, in all your diamond beauty, majesty, and dignity, ready to give all that you are to the work of service in the world.

Restorative Yoga Practice to Celebrate the Joy of Service

Restorative yoga is a practice that directs us inward to the place of peace within one's own heart and body. Our busy lives of service often become outer-directed and then we become chronically stressed. Restorative yoga poses heal stress with the grace of deep relaxation.

Unfortunately, few of us understand how to rest and relax. Most of us have become achievement-oriented. Living for the future, we can become anxious and exhausted trying to reach our goals. Relaxation involves letting go of striving and anxiety about the future and coming fully into the present moment.

In restorative yoga, we release effort, allowing ourselves to be fully supported and trusting the practice to hold us. Restorative yoga is a nurturing practice that embraces the receptive, feminine aspect of yoga, allowing us to be soft and vulnerable. This practice can be challenging to our goal-oriented minds. If we surrender to it, meeting any resistance that arises with tenderness and acceptance, we can learn how to compassionately care for ourselves.

B. K. S. Iyengar has refined certain yoga postures, with the subtle use of supports, to assist people recovering from illness or injury. These postures induce relaxation and renew health. Their physiological and psychological healing effects make them particularly beneficial during times of stress, exhaustion, illness, or injury.

Restorative yoga creates a deep state of physical and mental peace. Judith Hanson Lasater, PhD, PT, an unparalleled master teacher of this practice, writes that its benefits include releasing the spine, balancing hormone levels, nourishing the organs, bringing the nervous system into equilibrium, and renewing energy. Anyone interested in learning more about this practice should read her brilliant book, *Relax and Renew.*[18] Much of what is offered in this section originates from her inspired understanding of these poses.

A restorative practice is also a practice of *pratyahara,* the drawing in of the senses away from the distractions of the outside world so that we are able to listen to our inner voice, our intuition. Sensory input is registered but doesn't disturb the mind. We may remain aware of bodily sensation and thoughts, without identifying with or being swept away by them. We can notice the continual cycle of thoughts arising and subsiding without either pushing them away or becoming attached to them.

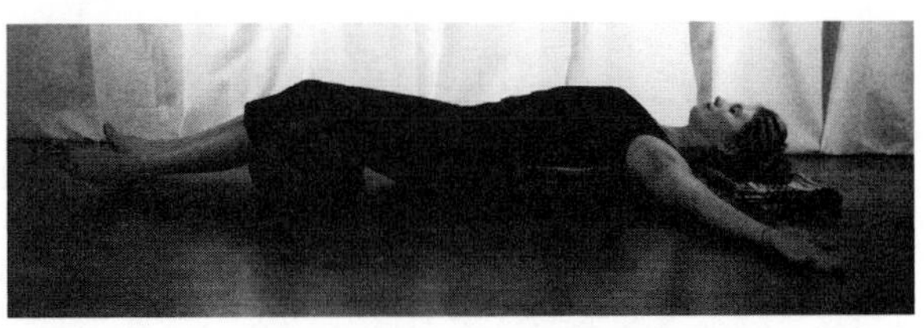

In this relaxed awareness, we witness that the thoughts arising aren't who we are, any more than the sounds emanating from a piano are the piano itself, as Judith Hanson Lasater describes. Just as we sometimes listen to music with our whole beings, in a restorative yoga practice we turn inward and listen with total attention, devotion, and concentration to the sensations of the body. We observe our inner world as both a vast fullness and an infinite emptiness. As we sink into the silence of a restorative pose, we are guided deeper and deeper inside, into the peace of the Self. As Rumi wrote:

> We search for Him here and there
> While looking right at Him.
> Sitting by His side, we ask
> O Beloved, where is the Beloved?
> Enough of such questions
> Let Silence take you to the core of Life.[19]

The silence of the restorative practice can lead us deeply into the Self, the source of effortlessly springing energy. There is nothing to *do* in a restorative yoga practice. Simply rest in the arms of infinite being, merging body and mind into its silence.

This immersion and renewal in the silence of the Self is especially important for Sacred Activists. From this wellspring of peace they will find restored hope, vitality, and energy to inspire their service in the world. In this practice we transcend the usual boundaries of personality and ego in order to experience our true interconnection with all life. From this interconnection, both natural compassion for others and the joy of a life of service are felt and renewed.

The Joy of Service Sequence: Restorative Yoga Practice

- Mountain Brook Pose
- Supported Bridge Pose – *Salamba Setu Bandhasana*
- Calves Supported on Cushion or Chair
- Legs Up Wall Pose – *Viparita Karani*
- Reclined Bound Angle Pose – *Supta Baddha Konasana*
- Supported Restorative Twist
- Supported Child's Pose – *Salamba Adho Mukha Virasana*
- *Savasana*

Mountain Brook Pose

In this pose the body takes the form of a mountain brook, flowing with ease over and around whatever it encounters on its path. Like water, the body flows effortlessly over gentle support under the knees, lower back, and neck.

Place one rolled blanket under your knees, one rolled blanket under the mid to low back from the bottom of the shoulder blades to the top of the sacrum, and a smaller roll under your neck. The head, tops of shoulders, sitting bones, and feet rest on your mat. An eye pillow will help the eyes to soften back. Turn your palms up, and let your legs release. Feel how the body gently flows up and down over the blankets, energy spreading evenly, with steadiness and ease. Rest here five to ten minutes. To come out, roll to your right side, resting a few more breaths.

Just sit there right now,
Don't do a thing
Just rest.

For your separation from God,
From love,
Is the hardest work
In this
World.

Let me bring you trays of food
And something
That you like to
Drink.

You can use my soft words
As a cushion
For your
Head.

—HAFIZ[20]

Supported Bridge Pose

Salamba Setu Bandhasana

In Supported Bridge Pose, the body is elevated from the base of the shoulder blades to the feet, while the tops of the shoulders and the head rest on the floor. In this gentle heart-releasing position, fatigue drains out of the legs as the space around the heart expands. Heart energy flows into the emptiness of the head; the mind settles. This is an excellent position for women on their moon-time or for anyone wishing to release tension.

Place two bolsters, folded blankets, or firm cushions length-wise down the mid-line of your mat. Lie back onto them so that your body is supported from the base of the shoulder blades to your feet, while the tops of your shoulders and your head rest on the mat. Your support should be high enough so that you feel a gentle curve opening the front of your chest. Lengthen your arms to the sides, palms turned up. An eye pillow helps the eyes soften. Receive the gentle nurturance that surrendering to this shape offers. Stay five to ten minutes, or as long as is comfortable.

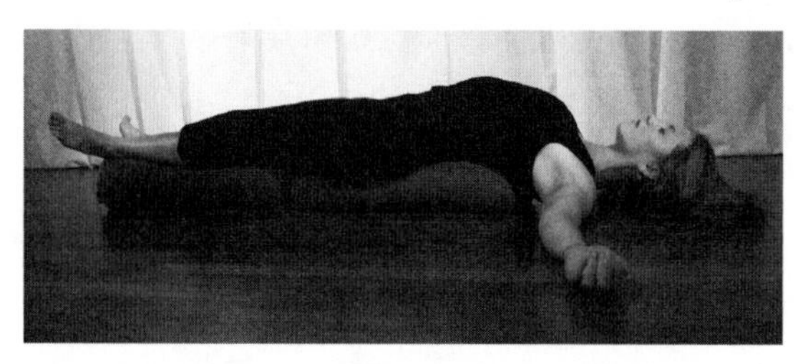

To come out of Supported Bridge Pose, slide back toward your head. Then roll to the right side, resting for a few more breaths.

Calves Supported on Cushion or Chair

After Supported Bridge Pose, rest your calves on the seat of a chair for a few minutes. To come out, slide back toward your head, and roll to the right side, resting for a few more breaths.

Legs Up Wall Pose

Viparita Karani

Legs Up Wall Pose is an important position for the Sacred Activist to practice, because it rests and restores the strong feet and legs that support our

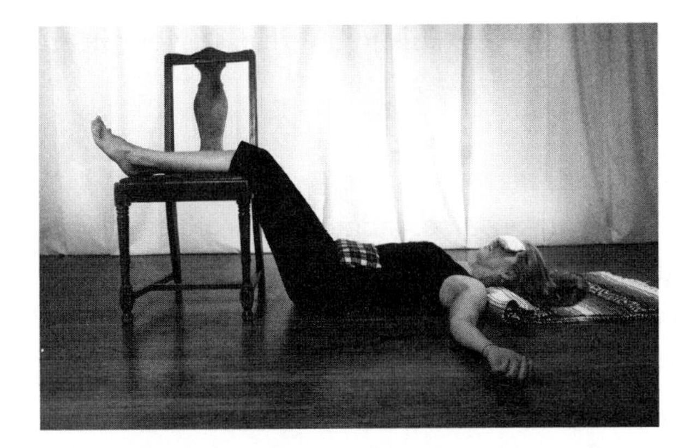

actions in the world. It gives us time to receive and renew, to let go of acting and giving, and to turn our compassion inward for a while.

Sit with one hip close to a wall, then swing around and put your legs up the wall. Your back can rest on the floor, or you can place a bolster or foam block under your hips and chest to elevate your hips slightly while your shoulders rest on the floor. This creates a gentle roundedness throughout your chest. If it feels like your chin is lifting too much, place a small pillow under your head and neck to support the curve of your neck, and adjust your forehead so that it's higher than your chin.

Spread your arms to the sides, opening your heart center, and turn your palms up. Release the tops of your thighbones toward the wall, softening your belly with each exhalation. If your legs or back feel uncomfortable, adjust the distance of your hips from the wall, or bend your legs slightly. An eye pillow softens the gaze inward.

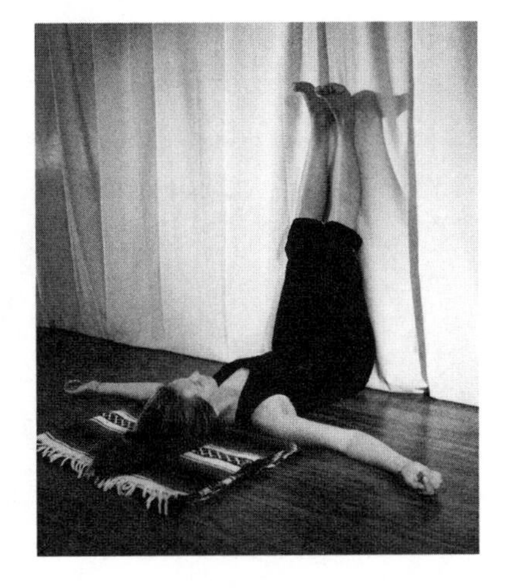

Observe how tension and tiredness drain down your legs, and energy flows like a waterfall into the quiet pool of your pelvis, brimming back into your heart and head. The breath releases your chest so that heart energy can flow freely in all directions, permeating your mind. Rest in this joy of release, your heart awake in pure love for all beings.

Reclined Bound Angle Pose
Supta Baddha Konasana

In this pose, the body is fully held so that it can completely relax in a position of openness. This is a deeply nourishing position for all those whose lives involve serving others and who are accustomed to giving rather than receiving. It is a powerful teacher of resting and opening, as the body and mind settle to their still source. Surrendering to the depths of the Reclined Bound angle Pose brings restoration and peace.

Fully supported, the body relaxes, and the mind can release and transcend the usual boundaries of personality. Beliefs, stories, and opinions melt away. The thought-waves of the mind resolve back into their source, and the Seer rests in the Self (Yoga Sutras I-2, I-3).

Set up a bolster vertically down the center of your mat, and place a folded blanket on the far end of it (this will be for your neck and head). Roll up two blankets and place them on both sides of your mat (these will go under your thighs). You can also place two rolled-up blankets or pillows on both sides of the bolster to go under your arms.

Sit in front of the bolster, drawing it up to your tailbone. Bring the soles of your feet together. You can strap them together if you like, or roll a blanket and place it over the feet and tuck it under your legs to hold your feet together. Open your knees to the sides, and let your thighs rest on the rolled blankets.

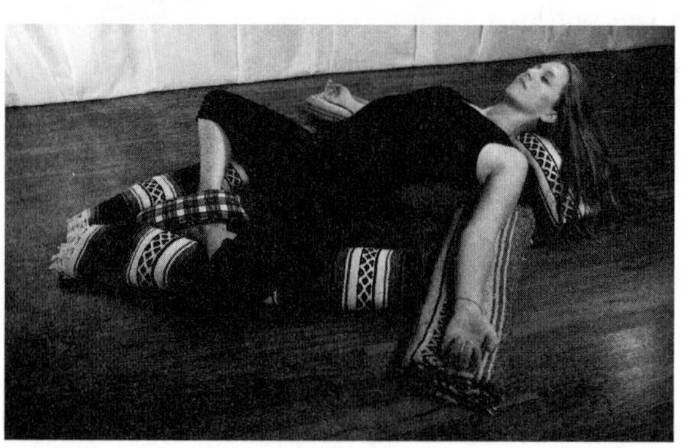

Lengthen your back down onto the bolster, placing your neck and head on the folded blanket. Adjust your props so that your forehead is higher than your chin; your chin higher than your chest; and your chest higher than your belly. Place an eye pillow over your eyes, and rest your arms on the center of the rolled blankets.

Sink back into your supports, allowing yourself to be held like a small child in her mother's arms. Watch the natural rhythm of your breath, and notice how as you relax your breath grows softer and slower. Your body and mind rock in the cradle of your breath. To quote Eckhart Tolle, "Feel yourself being an opening through which energy flows from the unmanifest source of all life through you for the benefit of all."[21] Rest as long as you like.

Slowly return when you're ready. Draw your knees together and lengthen your legs out, resting back on your bolster for a few more breaths.

Supported Restorative Twist

In this twist, the body drapes softly over the support, just like a blanket hangs over the edge of a bed. The front of the spine is fully supported, while the back releases into a gentle twist. There is nothing to do here—simply let go and surrender to the support beneath you, melting away all holding.

Kneel with your feet to the side of your left hip. Place a bolster or two folded blankets lengthwise, perpendicular to your right thigh. Put your hands on either side of your support. Inhale, and elongate your spine. Exhale, and slowly turn toward the right. With each inhalation, continue lengthening, and with each exhalation, continue turning, slowly unraveling the skin on your back and widening the wings of your kidneys.

Gradually ease the front of your spine onto the support, turning your head toward your knees. Your hands rest underneath the bolster, palms softly curled up. Let the unwinding of your spine invite your mind to dissolve, thoughts swirling away like leaves carried by a breeze. Sink into the earth and rest deeply for a few minutes.

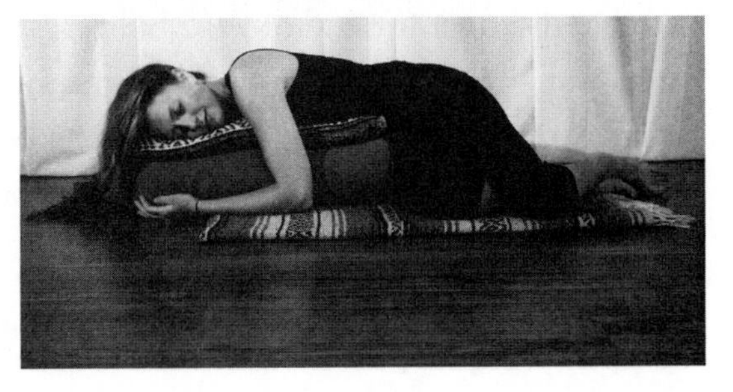

When you are ready, come to the other side by using your arms to support you as you inhale and rise up. Roll the knees to the other side, leaving the bolster where it is, and again gradually sink down into it. After an equal amount of time, slowly rise, widen the knees to either side of your support, and release forward into Supported Child's Pose (see below), with the front of your spine supported on your bolster.

Supported Child's Pose
Salamba Adho Mukha Virasana
In Supported Child's Pose, the front of the spine rests on a bolster or folded blanket(s). The body is held in the position of the child, surrendering for now all responsibilities, obligations, agendas, and roles that you carry in the outside world. Also release beliefs, judgments, opinions, and anything that creates an illusion of separateness. As you sink into the support of the earth, melt into the union that is the essence of yoga.

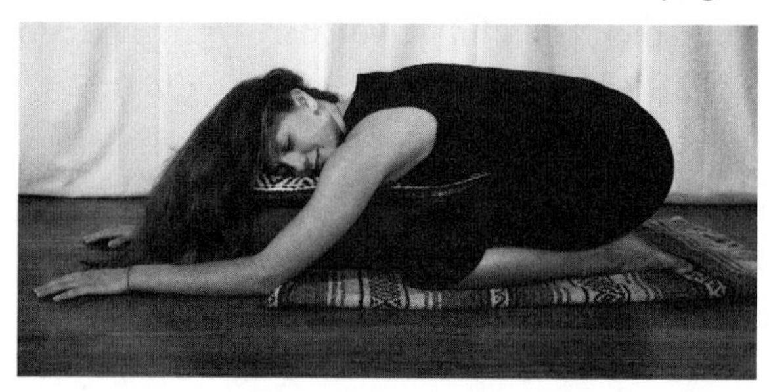

Kneel with a bolster or lengthwise folded blankets between your knees. You may wish to draw the bolster right up into your belly to support your spine as you hinge over. With your hands on either side of your support, inhale and elongate your spine. Exhale, and slowly release forward, folding deeply in the creases of your hips. Gradually settle the front of your spine onto the support. Rest your hands under the end of your bolster by your head, palms up.

Sink into the earth like a lover melting into the arms of the Beloved. Stay for a few minutes, then slowly unroll all the way back into *Savasana,* moving mindfully from the position of birth to the position of death.

***Savasana* for Restorative Practice**
No practice is more profoundly restorative than *Savasana,* or more impor-

tant for Sacred Activists to welcome into their lives. May its holy peace continue to initiate you into the all-renewing core of the Self, from where inexhaustible love energy flows forever.

Begin with your knees bent, feet flat on the floor. Gradually draw your awareness inward. Consciously and slowly, one at a time, lengthen your heels out along the floor, inviting your legs to fall back and rest.

Elongate your arms down to your sides, releasing any last vestige of stress or exhaustion. Turn your palms up into a soft, receptive position, like a baby's hands. Feel yourself letting go of whatever you have been holding onto.

Allow the skin of your face to soften away from the bones. Your eyes drop back in their sockets away from the inside of your eyelids. The gaze moves down, resting in the warmth of the heart. Vision now seems to come from your heart. Your ears also turn inward toward the heart, to listen to its whispering.

As you drop deeper and deeper into *Savasana,* your skin starts to grow more porous and transparent, almost translucent, so that the light inside you can radiate outward and the light all around you pours inward. As your skin continues to open to the light, your boundaries begin to soften and dissolve.

The boundaries of your personality also begin to release in *Savasana.* Let go now of anything that keeps you separate from other beings and from the joy and bliss of your essential nature, letting it all float away like clouds in the infinite blue sky.

From this vast awareness, find your breath and follow its path as it flows down into your body with your inhalation and as it empties out with your exhalation. Breathing in, your eyes soften; exhaling, your breath dissolves into emptiness. Breathe down into earth, breathe out into spaciousness.

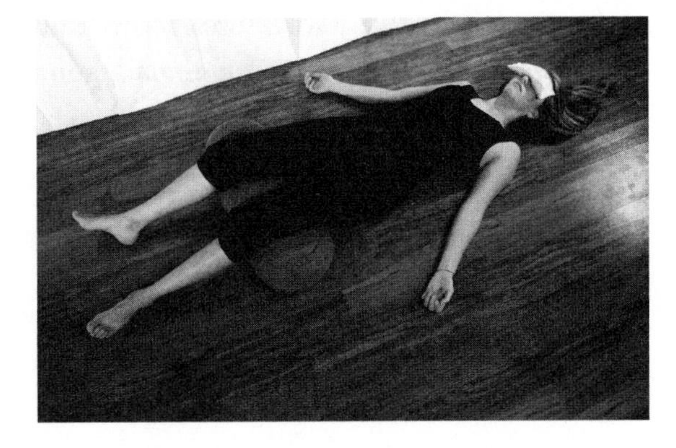

Notice the moments of stillness at the very end of the inhalation and at the very completion of the exhalation. This is not a holding but rather a suspension of your breath. Imagine this pause like a hawk suspended on a current of air. With the inhalation, drop down deep into the still pool of the pause at its end. Follow the exhalation all the way to its completion, and savor the exquisite moment at the end when it dissolves into space, like smoke disappearing into the sky. Inhale, and pause for a few heartbeats; exhale, and pause for a few heartbeats. Continue this practice for a few minutes.

Breathe into stillness, and breathe out into spaciousness, returning again and again to the breath, to the breath inside the breath. Breathe into the earth, the mother; breathe out to the sky, the father. Offer your body, mind, and heart on the altar of service. Expand and dissolve into the spaciousness of *Savasana.*

Let the spaciousness of the silence soak into every pore of your skin and every cell of your body. Let the silence take you to the core of your life. Rest in *Savasana* at least ten minutes.

When you feel ready to return from the spaciousness of *Savasana,* very slowly bring your awareness to your breath. Visualize your breath as a mist drifting toward you across a vast snowy field. Watch it flow into the core of your body, gently and tenderly touching the deepest places inside you. Imagine each inhalation is a blessing, and each exhalation is a prayer. Remember that this peace and stillness are always available to you, in any circumstance, simply by returning your awareness to your breath.

Grounded in this awareness, slowly begin your journey back from *Savasana.* Rise back up from *Savasana* gradually, like a deep-sea diver slowly returning from the watery depths. Pause when you want to pause. Remain connected to the beauty you experienced in the oceanic realms of yourself.

Let your transition back from *Savasana* be gentle, gradually coming fully into your body. Feel the warmth and radiance that surround your body, and the touch of the air on your face. Listen to the sounds around you.

When you are fully present in your body, in this moment, and this breath, roll to your right side, feeling the support of the earth beneath you. Slowly let your eyelids part, keeping your eyes soft, your brain quiet, and your heart open.

Feel how your soft compassionate presence radiates out from you. Imagine it cradling the whole world, and offer the benefits of your practice for the peace and liberation of all sentient beings. When you feel ready, sit up and bring your hands to the Namaste position in front of your heart.

Bowing to all beings, dedicate yourself to their sacred service. Inspired by the power of Heart Yoga, vow to embody the truth that all mystic sages of all traditions have expressed, here so perfectly stated by the modern Tibetan master Khyentse Rinpoche:

> Whatever circumstances arise, do not plunge into either elation or misery, but stay free and comfortable in unshakeable serenity . . . and just as the sun shines freely through space your compassion cannot fail to shine on all beings.[22]

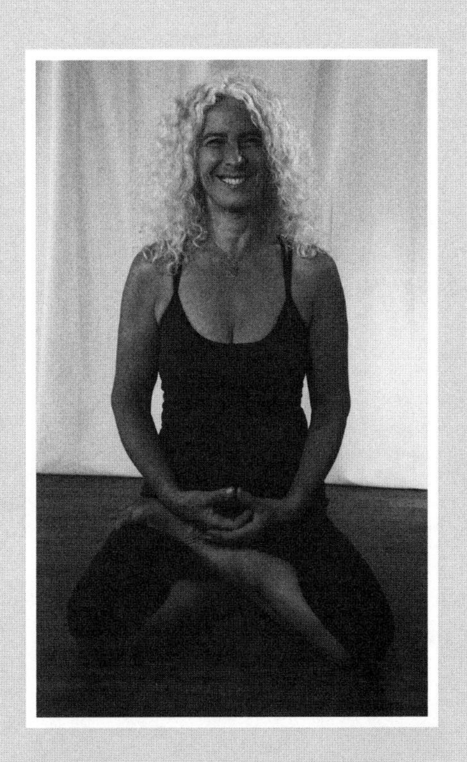

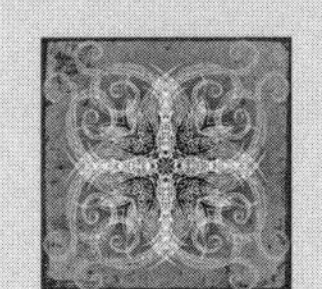 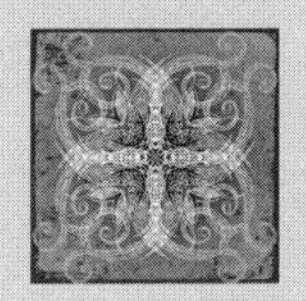 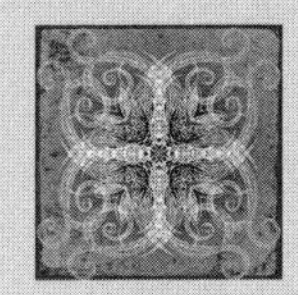

NINE
A Prayer

DIVINE BODY GOLDEN BODY

O, Divine Beloved,
Teach us
Moment by moment,
Stage by stage,
Illumination by illumination,
How most simply and richly
To unfold into union with you,
So that we may be revealed to ourselves
As you already know us:
Embodied souls, ensouled bodies—
Living flames of Incarnate Love
Fed incessantly by fountains of Eternal Fire
That keep streaming through us
From your burning sacred heart.
Awaken, Beloved, in each cell
The light-seeds you sprinkled there
Before the universe was created.
Let them ripen now
In tender golden harvest,
In this your hour of agony and of birth,
So that through us your all-healing vision
And holy compassion
Will flame out to renew the world.

—ANDREW HARVEY and KARUNA ERICKSON

19 July 2007

La Serpente Café, in the shadow of the Chartres Cathedral, France

Karuna's and Andrew's Journey to Heart Yoga

Karuna's Story

When I was a little girl, my grandmother, a mystical healer and a woman of irrepressible joy, would often say to me, "Remember, always, you are God's perfect child." Because I felt her unconditional love, her teachings sank deeply into me. It has taken me more than five decades to realize the fullness of her blessings.

Through my journey into the marriage of yoga and mysticism, I have begun to discover just how profound and far-reaching my grandmother's words are, not just for me but for everyone. My grandmother was a naturally holy woman who knew that we are all intrinsically blessed as embodiments of divine love and light, and that the meaning of life is learning how to receive this blessing in every dimension, and then express its truth as loving action in the world. Her life overflowed with joy. She often entered our house singing and dancing. She celebrated the announcement of the end of World War I by turning cartwheels around a fancy hotel lobby. Her last words to me before she died, said with a radiant smile glowing on her face, were "Let's go!"

I am starting to see how rich and potent is this experience of knowing ourselves to be the manifestation of the joy of divine energy. When we live this knowledge whole-heartedly, it transforms our lives and the world. The practice of yoga reveals and deepens this experience of the fusion of body and spirit. I am discovering how this union can lead to a subtle and profound evolution on the deepest cellular level, making accessible the new dimensions of courage, passion, stamina, and inspiration that are so essential at this crucial time in the world's history.

I humbly offer my experience, knowing that it is not unique to me but open to everyone, and has been at the heart of yoga philosophy from the very beginning. Four thousand years ago, the Vedic sages of India found "the treasure of heaven hidden in the secret cavern like the young of the bird, within the infinite rock." The "infinite rock" is, I believe, the cellular depths of the body. The "treasure of heaven" is the energy accessible to us when body and spirit marry. The "young of the bird" is the tender Divine Child, "God's perfect child," that this marriage births within us. The reclaiming of this ancient vision can transform our yoga practice, and our lives.

My journey into the mystery of my grandmother's teachings has had four stages. Many of you may have gone through similar stages in your unfolding journey. Sharing our stories to articulate these archetypal experiences acknowledges and magnifies their transformative power. I share my story in the hope that you will recognize aspects of your own story, and that it will inspire your continuing explorations.

First Stage

I had a happy and comfortable childhood in most ways. Growing up in a loving Jewish family in a comfortable suburb of Chicago gave me security and confidence. My grandmother was a constant inspiration. She taught me how to practice the mysteries of healing, to see the light in all beings, to feel the joy of life, and the power of love. When I was young, my father, a gentle scholar, held me on his lap as he read. He taught me devotion, concentration, and the value of prayer. My mother was a happy, energetic, and optimistic person who had trained to become an opera singer. She inspired me to have faith that I could do whatever I wanted to do.

Everything on the surface seemed perfect. Inwardly, however, my family and community were reeling from the shock and horror of the Holocaust. The wounds that this devastation dealt the psyche of my family gave me contradictory messages. On the one hand, I was taught that I had to succeed brilliantly in order to survive. On the other hand, my father used to warn me how dangerous it could be to be conspicuous in any way. All negative emotions were ignored, for they were too overwhelming to feel after what our culture had endured. I was trained to be relentlessly cheerful and positive at all times. My relationship with my body was ambiguous. While my family encouraged my athletic endeavors, I was always warned to be careful. Sexuality was never spoken of, and so became something shadowy and secret.

From these mixed messages I developed, like many of us brought up in the Western world, a false self addicted to intellect and success, and a sense of dissociation from my body. Outwardly I was successful, popular, and happy. Inwardly, I was a perfectionistic over-achiever, disconnected from my body. God's perfect child had developed somewhat of a split personality. My life has been a journey of healing this split of body, mind, and spirit.

Second Stage

Increasingly stifled by the protectiveness of my home, and longing for adventure, I decided with my partner Paul to move to San Francisco in the mid-sixties. It was there that I first discovered yoga in Ram Dass' seminal book, *Be Here Now,* so influential for many of my generation.

I started to practice the simple yoga poses that Ram Dass outlined. At this time, I was studying psychology at Stanford and Berkeley and was very intellectually oriented. Yoga awakened the cells in my body as if after a long sleep, helping to calm my restless mind. I encountered a copy of *Light on Yoga* by B. K. S. Iyengar and devoured it. What had begun as curiosity about yoga now began to crystallize into a life-long passion.

Meanwhile, it was the Vietnam War era, and in Berkeley the political climate grew steadily more menacing. Paul and I protested at anti-war demonstrations and were tear-gassed and chased by National Guardsmen with clubs. We saw people shot by police from rooftops, and protestors brutally beaten. This violence frightened and angered us, and we didn't know how to respond to it skillfully. Sometimes I wonder if my yoga practice had been more firmly established at this time whether I would have had then the courage and inspiration to know how to act effectively for political change.

Instead, Paul and I increasingly retreated into the calm and beauty of the nearby mountains to heal our spirits. As the political situation worsened, our hunger for a peaceful life in Nature grew, and we decided to move to the Yukon Territory in the Canadian wilderness. Fortunately, one of the few things I took with me from my old life was Iyengar's *Light on Yoga.*

Third Stage

Paul and I flew in a small plane into the majestic solitude of the Yukon, seventy-five miles from the nearest road. We lived in a one-room log cabin, settling in for a long Northern winter. Surrounded by mountains, lakes, moose, wolves, coyotes, eagles, and swans, everything I had been taught began to unravel. All that I had been doing in the Bay Area, like building a career, no longer seemed important. I wasn't sure who I was anymore, what I really wanted, or what was true in my life. After a few months of wondering if I was going crazy, I discovered that I only knew three things for certain: that I loved my partner, I loved to walk in Nature, and I loved practicing yoga.

Day after day I practiced, with deepening devotion and wonder. I started to experience the intertwining of my individual self with the Universal Self, as unveiled in the vastness of Nature around me. My body and mind moved toward the deep peace of their union. I began to understand more directly the words of the ancient yogic text, the Upanishads, "*Tat Tvam Asi,*" "I am That." Patanjali's teaching that the physical postures are "mastered when all effort is relaxed and the mind is absorbed in the Infinite"[1] started to feel more real and accessible. Sometimes I experienced my body as a dance of energy seamlessly interconnected with the energy dancing in all of creation. This brought me a joy I had never known before.

After almost a year, we left the isolation of the wilderness and moved to a serene and remote valley in the mountains of British Columbia, where we lived in a supportive and loving community and raised two children. After seven or eight years of practicing yoga on my own, I attended my first yoga class with Judith Hanson Lasater, PhD, PT, a renowned and loving yoga teacher. Judith's tender warmth, compassion, wisdom, and humor greatly inspired me. She encouraged me to share my practice with others.

I began to teach yoga and continued to study regularly with Judith and other inspiring teachers influenced by B. K. S. Iyengar, the great yoga master known for his genius in understanding the body. In the mid-eighties, I traveled to India to study with Mr. Iyengar directly.

I will always be grateful for the teachings of this great yogi. A new intelligence opened in my body as I began to integrate the subtle nuances of Iyengar's brilliant teaching. The fierce way he taught, however, scared me a little. I was drawn to a gentler way of practicing and teaching yoga, one that did not sacrifice any of Iyengar's precision and rigor, but married them to a more feminine approach. This softer approach, I intuited, could start to release me from my own perfectionism and harsh self-judgments, and begin to birth me into a more fluid, integrated, and loving relationship with myself.

I was next blessed to study yoga with Angela Farmer, whose soft yet strong and creatively experimental way of teaching delighted me and began to free me from my rigidity and the determination of my will. I then found these inspiring words from the ancient Taoist mystic, Lao Tzu, that became my guide:

> The typical way of people is to teach others to get rid of weakness and become strong, to remove softness and to become tough. However, the subtle Truth teaches to stop using force and become soft, to remove toughness and hardness and become gentle. Those under heaven who are soft can manage the strongest. Subtle energy has no form. Thus it can go into and out of any space. Therefore, I know the benefit of being soft and subtle and not using force. The learning of the subtle path is not only something that you know, but also something that you live. Many people know that not applying force brings greater benefit, but few are willing to do it. Living a life of no force is the subtle truth of Life.[2]

I started to dedicate my practice and teaching to "stop using force and become soft, and to remove toughness and hardness and become gentle." "Living a life of no force as the subtle truth of life" began to permeate my life. My practice of yoga deepened and began to reveal to me more profound realms of stillness and peace. My teaching became less preoccupied with detailed physical alignment, and more heart-centered and relaxed.

By the early nineties, however, I began to feel that both my yoga practice and my life had reached an invisible wall. The peace I had initially sought began to feel too comfortable. All the paths I had taken had been rich and rewarding, and I had been blessed with exceptional teachers. But still I felt restless and unsettled, as if I were missing something. There was something too isolated and protected about my life, and something too quiet and predictable about the yoga I was practicing. I yearned for an experience that could awaken me into a fuller life and a more active service to others. Without being able to articulate it, I longed to evolve my yoga practice and my life to marry peace with passion.

Fourth Stage

The thunderbolt I needed arrived in the form of Andrew Harvey's book, *Way of Passion: A Celebration of Rumi.* Rumi's divinely inspired poetry and Andrew's brilliant commentary awakened the fire in my heart. As I became more and more inspired and enraptured by Rumi's poetry, I began to feel the stirrings of sacred passion deep within my own heart.

> Passion burns down every branch of exhaustion,
> Passion's the Supreme Elixir and renews all things;
> No one can grow exhausted when passion is born!
> Don't sigh heavily, your brow bleak with boredom;
> Look for passion, passion, passion, passion! . . .
> Run, my friends, run far away from all false solutions!
> Let Divine passion triumph and rebirth you in yourself!
>
> —RUMI[3]

Rumi and Andrew challenged me into this rebirth with a fiery and urgent intensity. The inspirational mystical poetry of Rumi, Hafiz, and Kabir began to weave itself through my yoga practice and teaching. It infused the peace I knew with a new depth of ecstasy and passion, which I welcomed.

I was then blessed to study with two superb yoga masters, Patricia Walden and Rodney Yee, who both confirmed and richly expanded this vision of the potential of yoga to carry both peace and passion. Patricia Walden embodied exactly the marriage of precise movement with compassion and grace that I had been seeking. Her feminine wisdom deeply inspired me. Rodney Yee's creative use of imagery, combined with his readings of mystical poetry, further illumined and affirmed my experience of their potential to enhance yoga practice. Rodney's expertise in exploring the spiritual mysteries of yoga philosophy, as well as his extraordinarily nuanced understanding of the body's innermost subtleties, sparked my own quest to marry mystery with clarity. His heartfelt warmth suffused his teaching with loving generosity, encouraging me to move beyond my mind and open my own heart more deeply in my practice and teaching. Rodney's blend of feminine and masculine energies was a radiant example of the integration I was longing to embody.

I was eager to learn more about the realms of mysticism, and to integrate their ecstatic and passionate energy into my yoga practice. I began to hear glowing reports about the doctoral program at the University of Creation Spirituality in California, and when I saw that Andrew Harvey was one of the teachers, I listened to my heart and enrolled.

My first class at UCS was on Rumi, and Andrew Harvey was the teacher. Within five minutes, his wild and passionate presentation of the great Persian poet had tears rolling down my cheeks. Andrew's subsequent teachings gave me a vision of how I could connect with the fire of divine passion through devotion and longing, and how this fire could fuel the energy of service to others.

I loved Andrew's passion as well as his compassion, and his commitment to the expression of divine love as creative action, social justice, healing, and transformation in the world. I loved him, too, for not posing as a guru, but instead constantly stressing that all human beings have their own direct connection to God, and for cherishing and celebrating the gifts he saw in all the people around him. His teaching was totally in harmony with the teachings of my grandmother whispering in my heart. Andrew's tremendous energy and conviction was like a firecracker that woke me up from a peaceful dream, and helped me both to remember the core of divine consciousness within me and to live my life radiating from this remembrance.

In Rumi's blessing before Book IV of the *Mathnawi,* Rumi quotes the Andalusian poet Adi al-Riga, who said,

> I was sleeping, and being comforted
> by a cool breeze, when suddenly a gray dove
> from a thicket sang and sobbed with longing,
> and reminded me of my own passion.
> I had been away from my own soul so long,
> so late-sleeping, but that dove's crying
> woke me and made me cry. *Praise*
> To all early-waking grievers![4]

I was so grateful for Andrew's passion, which awakened my own. I was also a little afraid for him, because I sensed that his intense energy was not sufficiently grounded in his body, and I was concerned that he couldn't sustain the powerful energy flowing through him. As brilliant and mystical as Andrew was, like many of us it seemed that he wasn't living fully in his body.

One day, hesitantly and respectfully, I told him about my concern for him. I knew that he suffered from back pain and suggested that if he were more stable and steady on his feet, his back muscles would relax, and he would feel less pain. He welcomed my suggestion, and as he became more aware of how he was standing and rooted his feet in the earth, his back pain did lessen. He was thankful and asked me to teach some yoga postures in his classes, to help the doctoral students ground themselves and absorb the mystical teachings in the cells of their bodies.

We both began to see a new vision of the possibilities of yoga. Inspired by Andrew, I began to see more clearly how combining yoga with the passion of mysticism could deepen yoga's transformative power. Andrew, with my encouragement, began to see how being grounded in the body through devoted yoga practice could help the mystic embody mystical consciousness. We were both joyfully amazed by the synchronicity of our meeting, and at the natural interweaving of our two ancient paths. We were awed by the calm and exquisite truth of the path we found ourselves exploring together.

One day in a class on the Evolution of the Divine Human, Andrew played a CD of Jimmy Scott singing the theme song from the movie *Exodus*. I wept when I heard his heartbreakingly poignant voice singing these words, "This land is mine, God gave this land to me; this brave and lovely land to me." I felt then that the wounds of my childhood around the Holocaust were being directly healed, and that I could now, as a fully embodied human being, claim this earth, this "brave and lovely land" as my own. This was a moment of deep healing for me.

That night, the healing that had begun with Jimmy Scott's song continued in a yet deeper dimension. Awakening in the middle of the night from a dream, I found his words still running through my heart. This time I knew, with the stunned force of a revelation, that this "brave and lovely land" was also, in fact, my body. My grandmother had called me "God's perfect child," as were all beings. I experienced at that moment that my body was God's perfect gift to me—the divine's gift of embodiment to all beings. The energy flowing through my body felt both physical and spiritual, and I saw that any sense of separation is an illusion.

I felt my body radiating with divine beauty and holiness, united with all of creation. I felt the landscape of my body, its rounded hills and valleys, soft curves, moving winds, vast plains, flowing rivers and still pools, its forests and open skies. I knew directly that my body was the universe and the universe was my body.

I was moved to practice a few simple yoga poses, as if for the first time, and was amazed at the way they deepened the visionary experience. When old habits of self-doubt and self-judgment began to arise, I remembered a practice that Andrew had shared earlier that day. I visualized my grandmother floating lovingly above me, and I told her about the fears that were sabotaging me from awakening to my own God-given perfection. I imagined her extracting these fears from my body, like a magnet drawing up iron filings. As she did so, my body began to feel light and free.

This visionary experience continued to transform my yoga practice and teaching. A few months, later, Andrew and I began to teach a series of workshops celebrating what we had come to call the Sacred Marriage of yoga and mysticism. Andrew's vision of the marriage of the transcendent and immanent, masculine and feminine, body and soul, expressed itself in five great joys: the joys of transcendence, creation, love for all beings, the Tantra of tenderness, and service. In these workshops, Andrew articulated the vision of these joys, and I created yoga sequences that helped students directly experience and embody them. We were encouraged by the receptivity of our students to go more deeply into the mystery of the marriage, as they began to feel new levels of empowerment and freedom.

We continued to evolve and refine our work over the next few years. In an unforgettable week of teaching at Esalen, on the cliffs overlooking the wild ocean at Big Sur, all the aspects of the work that we had been honing came together and birthed a new level of awareness. Andrew and I began to further articulate the vision that informs this book. We spoke of the amazing potential that opens within yoga, when the practice and teaching of the asanas are combined with mystical imagery of the light-body from ancient traditions and esoteric anatomy. This felt like a powerful inspiration to us, and we evolved a teaching of the Sun Salutation with mystical imagery of the sacred centers of the light-body added to it. We were excited about the possibility of teaching all the yoga asanas from this perspective.

Having already had some experience of the cellular transformation that occurs when divine light is invoked into the body, we began to see how this new system would help us deepen and expand this transformation. By creating a precise and holy crucible for further engendering and grounding these experiences, this mystical yoga system would intensify and focus the light in a divinized body. Aurobindo and other great yogis had foreseen this as the next evolutionary step for humanity.

We investigated this vision and deepened our understanding of how the technology of transformation actually works. It is not as complicated as it may seem. The key to it is in the nature of the divine light. Just as physicists tell us that physical light is at once a wave and a particle, so the direct experience of divine light in the body is at once both an immersion in universal oceanic consciousness and a microscopic awareness of the light working with minutely precise intensity in every cell. As Rumi writes, "Do not think the drop alone becomes the ocean. The ocean, too, becomes the drop."[5]

As our practice of the yoga of the Sacred Marriage deepens, we find ourselves experiencing this vast expansion into universal presence as well as the microscopic attention to the minutest particles of the body. This fusion of universal consciousness with precise cellular awareness is the door through which grace can enter. It brings our whole being—mind, heart, soul, and body—into an ever-expanding unity and simultaneously gives us direct access to new levels of both profoundly calm and profoundly passionate energy.

This marriage of peace and passion, in turn, deepens, expands, and unifies heart, mind, spirit, and body. It creates an increasingly seamless, circular system of transformation. The absolute, the infinite, makes love to the relative, the finite. The finite, in responding to that love, fuses itself more intimately with its origin. This process, once awakened, becomes very simple and natural. With trust and openness to this practice, the divine light and grace do the rest.

Practice itself is the evolutionary crucible of divine humanity. Through practice, the immanent in us makes love to the transcendent, and through that lovemaking we open a pathway for the transcendent to love us into itself, as we embody transcendence.

Although I have practiced yoga consistently for over forty years, I often feel like a beginner on this subtle, demanding, and mysterious journey. Every practice brings new vision and new areas to explore. When periods of doubt, fear, or confusion arise, I need to stay grounded in my trust of the practice itself to realign me with awareness and courage, and to just keep practicing with an open heart.

A few years ago my life became nearly unbearable at times as my partner Paul struggled with and barely survived a series of major health crises.

I needed the strength, courage, stamina, and passion of a warrior to fight the limits of the medical system for Paul's life. I also needed the peace, trust, and practices of a mystic, such as prayer, breath awareness, and meditation, to weather the many dark nights of terror and loneliness without becoming numbed and paralyzed by despair. This descent into the shadows deepened my experience and understanding of the comfort and faith that yoga practice offers, and intensified my gratitude and sense of celebration of the wonder and joy of life.

Even after a lifetime's practice, I am awed at how completely the yoga practice we offer here provides a container to hold all of what I was asked to undergo. After experiencing so directly and nakedly how Heart Yoga, the yoga of celebration, can strengthen and inspire through even the most difficult times, I now know its truth and power in my cells and bones. I now can offer it confidently, understanding with my whole being that it provides you with tools you can use in your life that will sustain you through everything.

The yoga sequences we have created are not only both energizing and relaxing, they provide the foundation of peace and courage to help us continue to act from our deepest selves with focused compassion and kindness, whatever the challenges and circumstances. Heart Yoga keeps the psyche whole, as well as providing the fire and energy to go on acting and serving in the world even when everything seems to be falling apart.

What I want to share with all of you who find this book is the blessing of my grandmother as it has, through grace, ripened within me. Know that you too are God's perfect child, unimaginably cherished as you are, by a love that longs to help you evolve into itself. Trust that the Beloved you've been looking for your whole life lives within every cell of your own body. Trust also that as you open to the light and you work consciously with it, it will work consciously within you. It will unfold in you your true light nature, bringing you into the wonder of an ever-deepening marriage of all the seeming dualities with you, slowly turning you into alchemical gold. Be devoted, grateful, steady, and humble, practicing always with a beginner's mind. The great path of yoga, the *Mahas Patah* of the Vedas, the path of the Sun, will spring open to you. You will find the treasures of heaven hidden in the secret cavern within you, like the young of the bird within the infinite rock. You will discover yourself stronger and more serene than you ever imagined, able to embody and serve the light in all beings and in all circumstances.

> As the man and the woman in me
> unite in love,
> the brilliant beauty
> balanced on the two-petaled lotus
> within me
> dazzles my eyes.
> The rays
> outshine the moon
> and the jewels
> glowing on the hoods of snakes.
>
> My skin and bone
> are turned to gold.
> I am the reservoir of love
> alive as the waves.
> A single drop of water
> has grown into a sea,
> unnavigable.
>
> —LALAN[6]

I am grateful for this opportunity to share with you the divine child of inspiration that has been birthed from the marriage of yoga and mysticism in my life. My wish and blessing to you is that you celebrate the Sacred Marriage within yourself of passion and peace, masculine and feminine, immanent and transcendent; and from your own direct experience feel the birth of your creativity and passion, and of a commitment to become a channel of love and healing on our planet.

Andrew's Story

At the age of thirty-seven, after an awakening that revealed to me that all things are created and born from light, I had a startling encounter with the Dalai Lama. *Elle* Magazine sent me to interview him in Oslo in 1989, during the time he was to receive the Nobel Prize. At the end of two marvelous hours, I plucked up the courage as I was saying goodbye to ask him, "What is the meaning of life?" I shall never forget his roar of laughter at my question, and how he suddenly fell silent. He stared deep into my eyes, and said, in a loud voice that seemed to come from his belly, "The meaning of life is to embody the Transcendent." My whole being shook as he spoke. It was as if an electrical current passed up and down my body. I felt my body bursting with a strange new power that shocked me by its intensity.

In the weeks and months that followed, I found myself returning again and again to that moment of parting and to the Dalai Lama's answer. Nothing could have surprised me more, I realized. If His Holiness had said, "The meaning of life is to enter the Transcendent," or even "become One with it," I would not have been so strangely and marvelously disturbed. What he had said, however, was that it was necessary to embody the transcendent. My own experience, up to that moment, had been of the overwhelming power, glory, and bliss of the Divine Light. Now, I was being gently challenged to go beyond that awareness and somehow to bring the light down into my skin and bones and action. I was being asked to embody it and become, I now clearly saw that His Holiness had become, its humble living, breathing, grounded, utterly real and utterly authentic instrument. As I started to take in, in ever deeper ways, what His Holiness had said to me, I also began to uncover both the depths of what I came to call my addiction to Transcendence, and the psychological, biographical, sexual, and spiritual reasons for it.

I came to understand that my longings to vanish into the light, to drop my body altogether, to go beyond human relationship into what I imagined to be a far more ecstatic and transforming relationship with the One were in fact symptoms of a kind of dangerous, subtle illness. This illness, I recognized, had five main roots:

1. My early abandonment by my mother, who sent me away to boarding school at age six;
2. The brutal rigor of my English education with its disdain for physical weakness or vulnerability;
3. My early plumpness and lack of athleticism which led me to feel excluded from the camaraderie of sports;
4. An introjected and largely unconscious self-loathing that came from my awareness of my homosexuality;
5. My uncritical acceptance of the Judeo-Christian denigration of the body in favor of the soul and spirit, which I had found echoed also in the mystical traditions of Buddhism, traditional Hinduism, and Islam.

What the Dalai Lama awoke in me, then, was an increasingly precise critique of this addiction to transcendence, which I now noticed was shared by nearly all the seekers I met. Many of them were also possessed by the kind of subtly devastating split between body and soul that I had diagnosed in myself. I began to read Sri Aurobindo and Walt Whitman to try to heal this split, and pursued what I thought was a healthy sexual life to try to heal my self-rejection as a homosexual. These were, however, frustrating endeavors. Most of my friends were atheistic, and the majority of my lovers were either still subtly tortured by self-hatred or cheerful sensualists without a spiritual life. I could find no help either from the Indian master I was devoted to, for she obsessively stressed celibacy or heterosexual marriage as the path to God.

Then, in 1993, I met the great spiritual being who was to change forever my vision of the mystical path and the role of the body in it, Father Bede Griffiths. I met him when he was eighty-five years old, in the ashram he had created in South India, Shantivanam. I felt an overwhelming love for Bede. I felt, too, in his presence—in some way I could not understand but knew was real—that he was a living embodiment of the Christ. His heart was immense, his mind grand and supernaturally lucid, but what was most moving about him was the way his whole being, including his body, seemed to radiate the light of the humble majesty of his realization. I saw him one morning walking alone in the distance by the river Cauvrey, and for a moment it was as if he were a walking flame, a human fire angel.

I had come to meet him as part of a film crew that was shooting a documentary of his life. I had been asked to interview him. On the last day of filming, Bede took us all to a small dilapidated hut outside his ashram in the middle of gently swaying golden fields of corn. There, lying back on an old cot in his orange robes, supremely tender and relaxed, he spoke to me of the stroke three years before that had shattered his patriarchal dualism of body and spirit, and baptized him in a wholly new non-dual relationship with reality. He said, "What I realized after the stroke is that the body, too, must be transformed. The body, too, must be possessed and taken over and divinized in all its centers and desires by the Spirit. This is an immense, deep, slow rich work, and since my stroke it has been going on all the time. I feel that at every moment spirit and body are marrying within me more and more intensely. The spirit is constantly coming down, first through the center at the tip of my head—which the Indians call the *Sahasrara*—then through the heart center to every other center. It has entered by the sex region, also. I am rediscovering the whole sexual dimension of life, at eighty-five. A wholly new power of love has flooded me because of this. I find I love all beings more fully and tenderly, because my love is now in the body as well as the heart and spirit. Both Mother and Father, the Immanent and the Transcendent, are through grace integrating themselves within me. They are having their marriage within me and this inner marriage is birthing a wholly new being. The process isn't completely realized, and sometimes it is very bewildering, but when I get bewildered, I enter into silence and I allow the confusion to settle. Order comes out of chaos again and again. Increasingly, I find myself one with all things and beings; able to participate in the infinite beauty and bliss of the One appearing everywhere as the Many."[7]

Every word and gesture of that miraculous morning imprinted itself on my being, and I knew that I was being given the most accurate, candid, and exquisite teaching on how, without grandiosity or inflation, to embody the transcendent. After he had finished, I cried with gratitude. At last I had heard the whole truth from someone whom I loved with the whole of myself, and in a way that I could receive without any resistance and with all of myself on fire.

After filming ended I returned to Paris where I was living. I heard then that Father Bede had had a series of strokes and was dying. I couldn't bear not to see him again, so returned to India to spend two weeks with him as he battled in extreme suffering to stay alive. One night, as I sat by his bedside holding his hand, stricken by grief at how much he was going through and at the thought of losing my heart's Beloved so soon after having found him, he sat up suddenly, naked in bed. With his eyes streaming tears of bliss he said loudly, as if receiving dictation from another world, "Serve the growing Christ. Serve the growing Christ. Serve the growing Christ," again and again. Grace opened my mind and heart to hear the full glory of what he was transmitting. I knew that shattering pain and love was birthing Bede into direct prophetic consciousness. I knew that what he meant was that an apocalyptic time is the birth canal of a new kind of human being, the divine human, and that the time had come to give everything to serve its birth in humanity.

Bede, as a Christian monk, had used the word "Christ," but I knew he meant something far beyond any religious vocabulary. I knew, too, that "serving the growing Christ" would mean serving the growth of the divine human within myself, dedicating myself to birth divine love and divine knowledge, not just in my heart, mind, and soul, but also in the cells of my body as Bede himself had done. If I did not strive with all my being to serve my own growing Christ, how could I serve its birth in humanity?

After two weeks I had to return to France. Only a month later, I met the man, Eryk Hanut, with whom I was to spend the next twelve years. Bede had spoken frankly to me of how the spirit had entered his sex region. He had, in another conversation, given me what I knew to be a precise and succinct teaching on Tantra. With his hands in mine he had said, "Repressing sexuality does not work. It leads to bizarre and perverse behavior, as I have seen in many priests, monks, and aesthetics. Indulging sexuality does not work either; it leads to a kind of physical and psychic exhaustion. The only solution is to consecrate sexuality, to offer it wholly to the Divine, and to experience it as a form of Holy Communion."

In my marriage with Eryk, I was able to live at last this Holy Communion and to experience, in astounding depth and radiance, the all-healing and all-transforming power of Tantra. Since my body was blessed by the love of another, I was able at last to begin to bless it myself, and in fearless abandon to accept sexual rapture as a facet of the diamond of the Divine Ananda. Many times, as Eryk and I were making love, our bedroom would fill with Divine Light. I would see his hands, face, and body radiate green or golden light that is described in Tantric texts as the lights of the embodied sacred heart. From this holy experience I derived increasing strength, confidence, passion, and an abiding sense of the truth of ecstasy as the ultimate sign of the Divine Presence, and as the ultimate identity of the body itself.

During this time, I began to teach all over the world and especially in America. The message I was inspired to share was one that fused a tremendous sense of urgency about the world and its difficulties with a growing sense that the deep meaning of the death we are going through is that it is a necessary condition for the birth of a new kind of human being, one who humbly but passionately embodies the Transcendent.

For all the grace that had been given me, and for all my deepening experience of Tantra, I was still in many ways, disembodied and over-identified, although unconsciously, with the Transcendent. In 2000, when I was forty-eight, I had the great good fortune to have as a pupil in my Rumi class, Karuna Erickson. She had the courage to point out to me that while I was able to transmit sacred passion in my words and teaching, I was not embodying it completely. She perceived that I was in danger of burnout because I was not balancing passion with the radiant calm and fortifying peace that an illumined body could give me. I trusted her immediately because I knew her assessment was accurate, and did not come from any desire to denigrate what I was offering, but only to help me offer it from a more mature and integrated self, one that truly married transcendence and immanence and did not merely talk about it, however eloquently.

So began my adventure into yoga. I do not think I could have had a gentler and wiser guide than Karuna. Her compassion for my body has finally helped me to have compassion for it also. Her exquisitely profound understanding of the ancient tradition of yoga and its grounding in a living experience of the self has increasingly helped me to bring down the Divine Light into my skin, bones, cells, and feet.

What I have been able to offer Karuna, and I hope through her to the yoga community, is the marriage between physical yoga and the yogas of mystical ecstasy, visualization, meditation, and passionate energy that I had been working on for more than twenty years. Because Karuna and I so deeply trusted each other, we found that our experience and knowledge could fuse and merge effortlessly—in essence they came from the same source. Karuna had over many years experienced the source through her body. My search had led me through an increasing experience of it through my heart and mind. In our mutual love and work, grace could merge heart, mind, and body, and Heart Yoga, the yoga of celebration, was born, the Divine Child of the Sacred Marriage.

In the last seven years I have come to know, beyond any doubt, the following six things as a result of Heart Yoga.

1. The clue to the birth of the divine human lies not only in the awakening of heart, mind, and soul to the light, but in bringing down the light into the body and awakening the cells to the light in the body.
2. The most powerful path to this that I know is in the marriage of yoga and mysticism that Karuna and I have pioneered. The full impact of the marriage broke upon me gradually as Karuna and I dived headlong into the ancient mystical traditions of yoga and experimented with marrying yoga postures with mystical imagery and visualizations that worked directly with the transcendent light. Over time, I found that my whole being was being subtly opened to bliss energy, as if every cell were being kissed tenderly awake by the combination of the peace of yoga with the intense illumination of the Light.

3. As my vision of Sacred Activism has grown, I have had to transmit it in sometimes very difficult circumstances. My marriage collapsed, I lost all my money, but I had to keep on working incessantly under great psychological duress. Without the practices we share in this book, my being would have buckled under the demands. With the help of these practices, however, I was able not merely to survive but to refine my vision, to calm and ground it, and to find the inner and outer strength, peace and passion to embody it more and more authentically. The adventure into the marriage of yoga and mysticism turned into a necessity that I increasingly understood could inspire and ground others in our tremendously difficult times, as it had for me.
4. What became clear in the last years is that the great work of preserving the world, the work of Sacred Activism, cannot be done except by hearts awakened to love, minds instructed by wisdom, souls alive to their transcendent origin, and bodies increasingly supple to divine joy, divine energy, and the union of passion and peace that the marriage of yoga and mysticism makes possible. The world is not going to be saved by the guilty or desperate or the merely agonized. A new world can only be created by beings who know how to renew themselves constantly in the fires of the sacred heart and its radiation as bliss energy in the awakened body.
5. It is also becoming clear to me from my own daily and deep experience that the yoga we're sharing here is changing not only my body, which is becoming far subtler and far stronger, it is also deepening immeasurably my capacity to love all beings, to appreciate, savor, and adore the magic of divine beauty, and to go on, in hope and faith, pouring out my energies and vision to do what I can to help the world. In other words, I know there is a divine birth taking place in and through the great death that is everywhere destroying the old agendas and illusions, because through the grace of Heart Yoga and despite my own resistances, habits and failings, I am living this birth.

May all those who come to this book also be blessed by the Mother-Father, and learn through their grace how to marry the Immanent and Transcendent within themselves. May they be born peaceful and passionate, lucid and juicy, tender and exuberant, and completely committed in heart, mind, body, and soul to serving the creation of a new world from the ashes of the old.

> From joy all beings have come, by joy they all live, and unto joy they all return.
>
> —UPANISHADS[8]

NOTES

INTRODUCTION

[1] B. K. S. Iyengar, John J. Evans, and Douglas Abrams, *Light on Life: The Yoga Journey to Wholeness, Inner Peace, and the Ultimate Freedom* (Vancouver: Raincoast Books, 2005), p. 182.

[2] Andrew Harvey, *The Way of Passion: A Celebration of Rumi* (Berkeley, CA: Frog, 1994), p. 319.

[3] Dalai Lama, *The Universe in a Single Atom* (New York: Morgan Road Books, 2005), p. 110.

[4] Andrew Harvey, *The Way of Passion,* p. 139.

[5] Alan Jacobs, ed., *Poetry for the Spirit* (New York: Barnes and Noble, 2003), p. 473.

ONE

[1] Georg Feuerstein, *Teachings of Yoga* (Boston: Shambhala, 1997), p. 68.

[2] Andrew Harvey, *The Essential Mystics: Selections from the World's Great Wisdom Traditions* (New York: Harper San Francisco, 1996), p. 105.

[3] Ibid., pp. 64–65.

[4] Andrew Harvey, *The Return of the Mother* (Berkeley: Frog Books, 1995), p. 19.

[5] Octavio Paz, *Conjunctions and Disjunctions* (New York: Arcade, 1990), p. 77.

[6] Andrew Harvey, ed., *Teachings of the Hindu Mystics* (Boston: Shambhala, 2001), p. 82.

[7] Coleman Barks, trans. *The Essential Rumi* (New York: HarperOne, 1995), p. 107.

[8] William C. Chittick, *The Essential Seyyed Hossein Nasr* (Bloomington: World Wisdom, 2007), p. 220.

[9] Pandit Usharbudh Arya, *Yoga Sutras of Patanjali* (Honesdale, PA: Himalayan Institute, 1986), p. 62.

[10] Andrew Harvey, *Son of Man* (New York: Tarcher, 1998), p. 206.

[11] William C. Chittick, *The Essential Seyyed Hossein Nasr,* p. 88.

[12] Andrew Harvey, *The Essential Mystics,* p. 58.

[13] Andrew Harvey, *Perfume of the Desert: Inspiration of Sufi Wisdom* (Wheaton, IL: Quest Books, 1999), p. 53.

[14] Swami Adiswarananda, *Meditation and Its Practices: A Definitive Guide to Techniques and Traditions of Meditation in Yoga and Vedanta* (Woodstock, NY: Skylight Paths, 2003), p. 161.

[15] Ibid., p. 128.

[16] Ibid., p. 129.

[17] B. K. S. Iyengar, *Light on Yoga* (New York: Schocken, 1979), p. 31.

[18] Andrew Harvey, *The Essential Mystics,* p. 46.

[19] Ibid., p. 78.

TWO

[1] Dalai Lama, *The Universe in a Single Atom* (New York: Morgan Road Books, 2005), p. 111.

[2] William C. Chittick, *The Essential Seyyed Hossein Nasr* (Bloomington: World Wisdom, 2007), p. 220.

[3] Bruno Barnhart, ed., *The One Light* (Springfield: Templegate, 2001), p. 277.

[4] B. K. S. Iyengar, John J. Evans, and Douglas Abrams, *Light on Life: The Yoga Journey to Wholeness, Inner Peace, and the Ultimate Freedom* (Vancouver: Raincoast Books, 2005), p. 8.

THREE

[1] Andrew Harvey, *The Essential Mystics: Selections from the World's Great Wisdom Traditions* (New York: Harper San Francisco, 1996), p. 46.

2 Sri Aurobindo, *The Life Divine* (Twin Lakes, WI: Lotus Press, 2000), p. 1024.

FOUR

[1] Walt Whitman, *Leaves of Grass* (New York: Barnes and Noble, 2004), pp. 262–263.

[2] B. K. S. Iyengar, John J. Evans, and Douglas Abrams, *Light on Life: The Yoga Journey to Wholeness, Inner Peace, and the Ultimate Freedom* (Vancouver: Raincoast Books, 2005), p. 72.

[3] Daniel Ladinsky, *I Heard God Laughing: Poems of Hope and Joy, Renderings of Hafiz* (New York: Penguin Books, 2006), p. 38.

[4] Robert Bly, ed., *The Kabir Book* (Boston: Beacon, 1977), p. 17.

[5] Jnaneshwar, in Andrew Harvey, *The Essential Mystics: Selections from the World's Great Wisdom Traditions* (New York: Harper San Francisco, 1996), pp. 51–52.

[6] Robert Bly, ed., *The Kabir Book,* pp. 4–5.

[7] Jnaneshwar, in Andrew Harvey, ed., *The Essential Mystics,* p. 52.

[8] Coleman Barks, trans., *The Essential Rumi* (New York: Harper San Francisco, 1995), p. 279.

[9] Andrew Harvey, ed., *Teachings of the Hindu Mystics* (Boston: Shambhala, 2001), p. xxix.

[10] Rig Veda, in Andrew Harvey, ed., *Teachings of the Hindu Mystics,* pp. 5–6.

[11] B. K. S. Iyengar et al., *Light on Life,* p. 232.

[12] Ibid., pp. 232–234.

[13] Andrew Harvey, ed., *Teachings of the Hindu Mystics,* pp. 64–65.

[14] Andrew Harvey, *The Essential Mystics,* p. 85.

[15] Andrew Harvey, *Teachings of Rumi* (Boston: Shambhala, 1999), p. 3.

[16] Rumi, from Andrew Harvey, ed., *The Essential Mystics,* p. 162.

[17] B. K. S. Iyengar, *op. cit.,* p. 235.

FIVE

[1] Andrew Harvey, ed., *Teachings of the Hindu Mystics* (Boston: Shambhala, 2001), p. 17.

[2] Ibid., p. 62.

[3] Andrew Harvey, *The Way of Passion: A Celebration of Rumi* (Berkeley: Frog Books, 1994), p. 215.

[4] Ibid., p. 31.

[5] Ibid., p. 40.

[6] Ibid., p. 164.

[7] Ibid.

[8] Ibid., p. 132.

[9] Ibid., p. 110.

[10] Pandit Usharbudh Arya, *Yoga Sutras of Patanjali* (Honesdale, PA: Himalayan Institute, 1986), pp. 93 & 114.

[11] Andrew Harvey, *The Way of Passion,* p. 318.

[12] Andrew Harvey, *op. cit.,* p. 138.

[13] Daniel Ladinsky, *I Heard God Laughing: Poems of Hope and Joy, Renderings of Hafiz,* (New York: Penguin Books, 2006), p. 38.

SIX

[1] Walt Whitman, *Leaves of Grass* (New York: Barnes and Noble, 2004), p. 211.

[2] Ibid., preface.

[3] Andrew Harvey, ed., *Teachings of the Hindu Mystics* (Boston: Shambhala, 2001), p. 96.

[4] Andrew Harvey, *Light Upon Light: Inspirations from Rumi* (Berkeley: North Atlantic Books, 1996), p. 185.

[5] Daniel C. Matt, *The Essential Kabbalah* (New York: HarperOne, 1996), p. 99.

[6] Andrew Harvey, ed., *Teachings of the Hindu Mystics,* p. 95.

[7] Andrew Harvey, *The Essential Mystics, Selections from the World's Great Wisdom Traditions* (New York: Harper San Francisco, 1996), pp. 4–5.

[8] Marcus Braybrooke, ed., *The Bridge of Stars* (London: Thorsons, 2001), p. 49.

[9] Ibid., p. 212.

[10] Andrew Harvey, *The Essential Mystics,* pp. 74–75.

[11] Andrew Harvey, ed., *Teachings of the Hindu Mystics,* pp. 32–33.

[12] Andrew Harvey, *The Essential Mystics,* p. 15.

[13] Robert Bly, *The Kabir Book* (Boston: Beacon, 1977), p. 35.

[14] Andrew Harvey, *The Essential Mystics,* pp. 3–4.

[15] Marcus Braybrooke, ed., *The Bridge of Stars,* p. 69.

[16] Andrew Harvey, ed., *Teachings of the Hindu Mystics,* p. 10.

SEVEN

[1] Alistair Shearer, trans., *Effortless Being: The Yoga Sutras of Patanjali* (New York: HarperCollins, 1990), p. 61.

[2] B. K. S. Iyengar, John J. Evans, and Douglas Abrams, *Light on Life: The Yoga Journey to Wholeness, Inner Peace, and the Ultimate Freedom* (Vancouver: Raincoast Books, 2005), p. 59.

[3] Ibid.

[4] Walt Whitman, *Leaves of Grass* (New York: Barnes and Noble, 2004).

[5] Andrew Harvey, ed., *Teachings of the Hindu Mystics* (Boston: Shambhala, 2001), p. 21.

[6] B. K. S. Iyengar, *op. cit.,* p. 59.

[7] Marcus Braybrooke, ed., *The Bridge of Stars* (London: Thorsons, 2001), p. 149.

[8] Daniel Ladinsky, ed., *The Gift* (New York: Penguin Compass, 1999), p. 277.

[9] Derek Walcott, *Collected Poems* (New York: Noonday Press, 1984), p. 328.

[10] Marcus Braybrooke, ed., *The Bridge of Stars,* p. 131.

[11] Ibid., p. 126.

[12] B. K. S. Iyengar, *op. cit.,* p. 62.n.

[13] Andrew Harvey, *The Way of Passion: A Celebration of Rumi* (Berkeley: Frog Books, 1994), pp. 317–318.

[14] Ibid., p. 94.

[15] Ibid., p. 314.

[16] Marcus Braybrooke, *The Bridge of Stars,* p. 125.

[17] Ibid., p. 101.

[18] Daniel Ladinsky, *I Heard God Laughing: Poems of Hope and Joy, Renderings of Hafiz,* (New York: Penguin Books, 2006), p. 38.

EIGHT

[1] Walt Whitman, *Leaves of Grass* (New York: Barnes and Noble, 2004), pp. 32–33.

[2] Daniel C. Matt, *The Essential Kabbalah* (San Francisco: Harper San Francisco, 1996), p. 155.

[3] Ibid., p. 15.

[4] Andrew Harvey, *Teachings of Rumi* (Boston: Shambhala, 1999), p. 88.

[5] Andrew Harvey, *The Essential Mystics, Selections from the World's Great Wisdom Traditions* (New York: Harper San Francisco, 1996), p. 94.

[6] Ibid., pp. 50–51.

[7] Andrew Harvey, ed., *Teachings of the Hindu Mystics* (Boston: Shambhala, 2001), p. xxix.

[8] Richard Freeman, *The Yoga Matrix,* audio set (Louisville, CO: Sounds True, 2003).

[9] Andrew Harvey, *The Essential Mystics,* p. 163.

[10] Coleman Barks, trans., *The Essential Rumi* (New York: HarperOne, 1995), p. 109.

[11] Marcus Braybrooke, ed., *The Bridge of Stars* (London: Thorsons, 2001), p. 57.

[12] Coleman Barks, trans., *The Essential Rumi,* p. 105.

NINE

[1] Andrew Harvey, *Light Upon Light: Inspirations from Rumi* (Berkeley: North Atlantic Books, 1996), p. 233.

[2] Andrew Harvey, *The Essential Mystics: Selections from the World's Great Wisdom Traditions* (New York: Harper San Francisco, 1996), p. 100.

[3] Andrew Harvey, ed., *Teachings of the Hindu Mystics* (Boston: Shambhala, 2001), p. 15.

[4] Steven Larsen, *A Fire in the Mind* (New York: Anchor, 1992), p. 238.

[5] Andrew Harvey, unpublished translation.

[6] Jack Kornfield, *The Wise Heart: A Guide to the Universal Teachings of Buddhist Psychology* (New York: Bantam, 2008), p. 355.

[7] See www.joannamacy.com.

[8] Quoted in *Unity Magazine,* Missouri: Unity Village, www.unitymagazine.org, Jan-Feb 2010, p. 14.

[9] B. K. S. Iyengar, John J. Evans, and Douglas Abrams, *Light on Life: The Yoga Journey to Wholeness, Inner Peace, and the Ultimate Freedom* (Vancouver: Raincoast Books, 2005), p. x.

[10] Ibid.

[11] Ibid.

[12] Marcus Braybrooke, ed., *The Bridge of Stars* (London: Thorsons, 2001), p. 31.

[13] Andrew Harvey, *The Essential Mystics,* pp. 192–193.

[14] Ibid., p. 44.

[15] Marcus Braybrooke, ed., *The Bridge of Stars,* p. 126.

[16] B. K. S. Iyengar et al., *Light on Life,* p. 62.n.

[17] Andrew Harvey, *The Way of Passion: A Celebration of Rumi* (Berkeley, CA: Frog Books, 1994), pp. 317–318.

[18] Judith Hanson Lasater, PhD, PT, *Relax and Renew* (Berkeley: Rodmell Press, 1995).

[19] Andrew Harvey, *The Way of Passion.*

[20] Daniel Ladinsky, ed., *The Gift* (New York: Penguin Compass, 1999), p. 183.

[21] Eckhart Tolle, *A New Earth* (New York: Penguin, 2005), p. 305.

[22] Mathieu Ricard, *Journey to Enlightenment* (New York: Aperture Press, 1997), p. 41.

KARUNA'S AND ANDREW'S JOURNEY TO HEART YOGA

[1] Alistair Shearer, trans., *Effortless Being: The Yoga Sutras of Patanjali* (New York: HarperCollins, 1990), p. 83.

[2] Lao Tzu, *Tao Te Ching,* trans. by Jonathan Star (New York: Tarcher/Penguin, 2001), chapters 78 and 10.

[3] Andrew Harvey, *Teachings of Rumi* (Boston: Shambhala, 1999), p. 88.

[4] Coleman Barks, trans., *The Essential Rumi* (New York: HarperOne, 1995), pp. xvi–xvii.

5 Andrew Harvey, The Way of Passion: A Celebration of Rumi (Berkeley, CA: Frog Books, 1994), p. 215.

[6] Andrew Harvey, ed., *Teachings of the Hindu Mystics* (Boston: Shambhala, 2001), p. 94.

[7] Andrew Harvey, *Sun at Midnight* (New York: Tarcher, 2002).

[8] Andrew Harvey, *The Essential Mystics: Selections from the World's Great Wisdom Traditions* (New York: Harper San Francisco, 1996), p. 37.

BIBLIOGRAPHY

Sri Aurobindo. *The Life Divine*. Twin Lakes, WI: Lotus Press, 2000.

Sri Aurobindo. *The Synthesis of Yoga*. Pondicherry, India: Sri Aurobindo Ashram, 2000.

Arya, Pandit Usharbudh. *Yoga Sutras of Patanjali*. Honesdale, PA: Himalayan Institute, 1986.

Balaskis, Janet. *Preparing for Birth with Yoga*. London: Element Books, 1994.

Barks, Coleman, trans. *The Essential Rumi*. New York: HarperOne, 1995.

Barnhart, Bruno, ed. *The One Light*. Springfield: Templegate, 2001.

Bly, Robert, ed. *The Kabir Book*. Boston: Beacon, 1977.

Braybrooke, Marcus, ed. *The Bridge of Stars*. London: Thorsons, 2001.

Calais-Germain, Blandine. *Anatomy of Movement (Revised Edition)*. Seattle: Eastland Press, 2007.

Chittick, William C. *The Essential Seyyed Hossein Nasr*. Bloomington: World Wisdom, 2007.

Chödrön, Pema. *The Wisdom of No Escape and the Path of Loving Kindness*. Boston: Shambhala, 2001.

Cope, Stephen. *Yoga and the Quest for the True Self*. New York: Bantam, 2000.

Coulter, H. David. *Anatomy of Hatha Yoga: A Manual for Students, Teachers and Practitioners*. Indianapolis: Body and Breath, 2001.

Dalai Lama. *The Universe in a Single Atom*. New York: Morgan Road, 2005.

Desikachar, T. K. V. *The Heart of Yoga: Developing a Personal Practice*. Rochester: Inner Traditions, 1999.

Farhi, Donna. *Teaching Yoga: Exploring the Teacher-Student Relationship*. Berkeley: Rodmell Press, 2006.

Farhi, Donna. *The Breathing Book: Vitality & Good Health Through Essential Breath Work*. New York: Holt Paperbacks, 1996.

Feuerstein, Georg. *The Yoga Sutras of Patanjali: A New Translation and Commentary*. Rochester: Inner Traditions, 1989.

Feuerstein, Georg. *Teachings of Yoga*. Boston: Shambhala, 1997.

Freeman, Richard. *The Yoga Matrix* (audio). Louisville, CO: Sounds True, 2003.

Harvey, Andrew. *Light Upon Light: Inspirations from Rumi.* Berkeley, CA: North Atlantic Books, 1996.

Harvey, Andrew. *Sun at Midnight.* New York: Tarcher, 2002.

Harvey, Andrew. *The Direct Path: Creating a Personal Journey to the Divine Using the World's Spiritual Traditions.* New York: Broadway, 2001.

Harvey, Andrew. *The Essential Mystics: Selections from the World's Great Wisdom Traditions.* New York: Harper San Francisco, 1996.

Harvey, Andrew. *The Return of the Mother.* Berkeley, CA: Frog Books, 1995.

Harvey, Andrew. *Son of Man.* New York: Tarcher, 1998.

Harvey, Andrew. *The Hope.* New York: Hay House, 2009.

Harvey, Andrew. *Perfume of the Desert: Inspiration of Sufi Wisdom.* Wheaton, IL: Quest Books, 1999.

Harvey, Andrew, ed. *Teachings of the Hindu Mystics.* Boston: Shambhala, 2001.

Harvey, Andrew. *Teachings of Rumi.* Boston: Shambhala, 1999.

Harvey, Andrew. *The Way of Passion: A Celebration of Rumi.* Berkeley, CA: Frog, 1994.

Iyengar, B. K. S., Evans, John J., and Abrams, Douglas. *Light on Life: The Yoga Journey to Wholeness, Inner Peace, and the Ultimate Freedom.* Vancouver: Raincoast Books, 2005.

Iyengar, B. K. S. *Light on Pranayama: The Yogic Art of Breathing.* New York: The Crossroad Publishing Company, 1981.

Iyengar, B. K. S. *Light on the Yoga Sutras of Patanjali.* Ottawa: Educa Books, 1993.

Iyengar, B. K. S. *Light on Yoga.* New York: Schocken, 1979.

Iyengar, B. K. S. *The Tree of Yoga.* Boston: Shambhala, 2002.

Jacobs, Alan, ed. *Poetry for the Spirit.* New York: Barnes and Noble, 2003.

Kornfield, Jack. *A Path with Heart: A Guide Through the Perils and Promises of Spiritual Life.* New York: Bantam, 1993.

Kornfield, Jack. *The Wise Heart: A Guide to the Universal Teachings of Buddhist Psychology.* New York: Bantam, 2008.

Daniel, Ladinsky. *I Heard God Laughing: Poems of Hope and Joy, Renderings of Hafiz* (New York: Penguin Books, 2006), p. 38.Ladinsky, Daniel, Mindlin, Henry S., and Wilberforce Clarke, H., eds. *I Heard God Laughing: Renderings of Hafiz*. Walnut Creek, CA: Sufism Reoriented, 1996.

Ladinsky, Daniel, ed. *The Gift*. New York: Penguin Compass, 1999.

Ladinsky, Daniel, ed. *The Subject Tonight is Love: 60 Wild and Sweet Poems of Hafiz*. Myrtle Beach, SC: Pumpkin House Press, 1996.

Larsen, Steven. *A Fire in the Mind*. New York: Anchor, 1992.

Lasater, Judith. *Living Your Yoga*. Berkeley, CA: Rodmell Press, 1999.

Lasater, Judith. *Relax and Renew*. Berkeley, CA: Rodmell Press, 1995.

Lee, Diane. *The Pelvic Girdle*. Philadelphia: Churchill Livingstone, 2004.

Levine, Stephen. *Healing into Life and Death*. New York: Anchor, 1989.

Long, Ray. *The Key Muscles of Hatha Yoga*. Plattsburgh: BandhaYoga, 2009.

Matt, Daniel C. *The Essential Kabbalah*. New York: HarperOne, 1996.

Miller, Barbara Stoller. *Yoga: Discipline of Freedom*. New York: Bantam, 1998.

Nikhilananda, Swami. *The Gospel of Sri Ramakrishna*. New York: Ramakrishna-Vivekananda Center, 1958.

Maharaj, Nisargadatta, Sudhaker S. Dikshit. ed., and Maurice Frydmann, trans. *I Am That: Talks with Sri Nisargadatta*. Durham, NC: Acorn Press, 1999.

Olsen, Andrea. *BodyStories: A Guide to Experiential Anatomy*. Lebanon, NH: UPNE, 2004.

Paz, Octavio. *Conjunctions and Disjunctions*. New York: Arcade, 1990.

Prabhavananda, Swami, and Isherwood, Christopher. *How to Know God: The Yoga Aphorisms of Patanjali*. Hollywood: Vendanta Press, 1983.

Ricard, Mathieu. *Journey to Enlightenment*. New York: Aperture Press, 1997.

Rosen, Richard. *Yoga of Breath*. Berkeley, CA: Shambhala, 2002.

Salzberg, Sharon. *Lovingkindness: The Revolutionary Art of Happiness*. Berkeley, CA: Shambhala, 1997.

Sat Prem. *Sri Aurobindo or the Adventure of Consciousness*. Faridabad, India: Thomson Press, 2000.

Schatz, Mary Pullig, Iyengar, B. K. S., and Connor, William. *Back Care Basics*. Berkeley: Rodmell Press, 1992.

Schiffmann, Erich. *Yoga: the Spirit and Practice*. New York: Pocket, 1996.

Shearer, Alistair. *Effortless Being: The Yoga Sutras of Patanjali.* New York: HarperCollins, 1990.

Starhawk. *The Spiral Dance: A Rebirth of the Ancient Religion of the Goddess: 20th Anniversary Edition.* New York: HarperOne, 1999.

Suzuki, Shunruyu. *Zen Mind, Beginner's Mind.* New York: Random House Inc, 1972.

Svatmarama. *The Hatha Yoga Pradipika.* Woodstock, NY: YogaVidya, 2002.

Swami Adiswarananda. *Meditation and Its Practices: A Definitive Guide to Techniques and Traditions of Meditation in Yoga and Vedanta.* Woodstock, NY: Skylight Paths, 2003.

Swenson, David. *Ashtanga Yoga: The Practice Manual.* Austin, TX: Ashtanga Yoga Productions, 2000.

Taimni, I. K. *The Science of Yoga: The Yoga Sutras of Patanjali in Sanskrit.* Wheaton, IL: Quest Books, 1961.

Tolle, Eckhart. *A New Earth.* New York: Penguin, 2005.

Vaughn-Lee, Llewellyn. *Love is a Fire.* Point Reyes Station, CA: The Golden Sufi Center, 2000.

Walcott, Derek. *Collected Poems.* New York: Noonday Press, 1984.

Whitman, Walt. *Leaves of Grass.* New York: Barnes and Noble, 2004.

Yee, Rodney, and Zolotow, Nina. *Yoga: The Poetry of the Body.* St. Martin's Griffin: New York, 2002.

Yee, Rodney. *Moving into Balance: 8 Weeks of Yoga with Rodney Yee.* Emmaus, PA: Rodale Books, 2004.

ACKNOWLEDGMENTS

To all the inspired teachers who have seen the sacred importance of our vision and championed it so generously.

To all our students over the years whose enthusiasm and feedback have encouraged us immeasurably.

To Ned Leavitt for his advocacy of our book.

To Richard Grossinger for having the fearlessness to publish this book.

To Hisae Matsuda for her lovely presence and tireless help.

To Kathy Glass for her scrupulous and imaginative copyediting.

To Jill Angelo, wonderful friend and executive director of the Institute of Sacred Activism.

—Karuna and Andrew

I feel so much appreciation for my dear friend, brother, and fellow traveler, Andrew. This book would not have been birthed without your vision, passion, genius, and love. My greatest teacher has been my grandmother, who has guided and inspired me with her loving and joyful spirit throughout my life. I'm deeply grateful for the wisdom of B. K. S. Iyengar, Baba Hari Das, Ram Dass, Judith Hanson Lasater, Rodney Yee, Caroline Myss, along with numerous other teachers I've been fortunate enough to encounter along my path. I've been so blessed and inspired by the company of many brilliant and loving students over the past forty years. Huge thanks to my incredible friends, for their love, compassion, kindness, and insight: Mary, Diane, Rosalyn, Jordanna, Norah, Duncan, Terence, Pamela, Ilene, Maureen, Suz, Susan, Ally, and so many others, thank you. I'm eternally thankful for the continuous loving support of the circle of my ancestors, whom I often feel around me. My family has always been there for me: Doris, Fred, Mark, Ellen, Paula, Eric, Janet, Steven—thank you. Immense gratitude to Ricardo for his beautiful photos, infinite patience, loving heart, and making me laugh; and to Eliza, Callie, Yogita, and Richard for being such graceful and willing models, as well as true friends. Heartfelt thanks to my children, Amanda, Eli, and Mosang, for seeing my gifts when I was unsure, for believing in me and always being there to help with their wisdom, kindness, and clarity. I feel so blessed by your support and so grateful for our deep connection and love. Inexpressible gratitude to Paul, the love of my life for more than forty-five years . . . the wind beneath my wings . . . for his faith and endless tender compassion; for being willing to open his heart to me over and over again. . . . And blessings to my grandson Lucero for his joyful inspiration and radiant smile. May this book bring greater peace, ease, healing, and love into the world.

—Karuna

To all the teachers who have guided us, especially His Holiness the Dalai Lama and father Bede Griffiths.

To Nancy Koppelmann for giving me hope.

To Sheryl Leach and Howard Rosenfeld for their endless generosity and sweetness of heart.

—Andrew

ABOUT THE AUTHORS

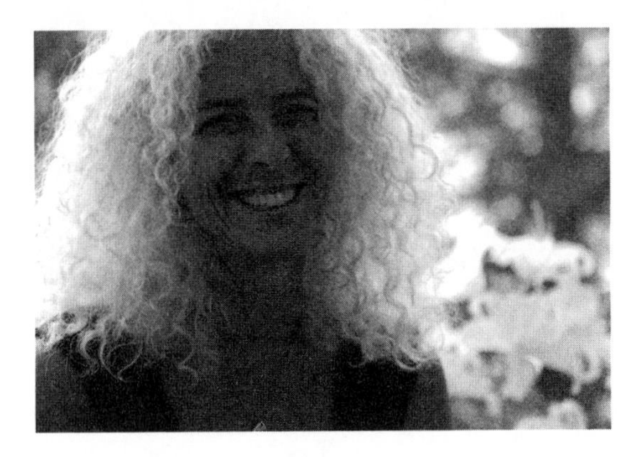

Karuna Erickson has lived in the mountains of British Columbia with her husband for forty years. She has been a devoted yoga teacher and psychotherapist since 1970. She received her bachelor's degree from Stanford University and a Master's in Social Work from the University of California, Berkeley. Erickson is the director of the Heart Yoga Center, a registered yoga teacher training school with Yoga Alliance (www.yogaalliance.org). She has trained many yoga teachers for over twenty years and teaches yoga internationally, interweaving Sufi poetry and Buddhist practices of mindfulness and loving-kindness meditation into her classes. She leads annual retreats, yoga-teacher trainings, and workshops in Canada, the U.S., Bali, and Costa Rica. Erickson also teaches courses with Andrew Harvey internationally. She has assisted Rodney Yee (www.yeeyoga.com) and Judith Hanson Lasater (www.judithlasater.com) in yoga workshops and considers them, along with B. K. S. Iyengar, to be her most influential teachers.

For Karuna Erickson's teaching schedule, for other information, or to contact her to book a workshop, visit www.yogakaruna.com or write her at erickson@netidea.com.

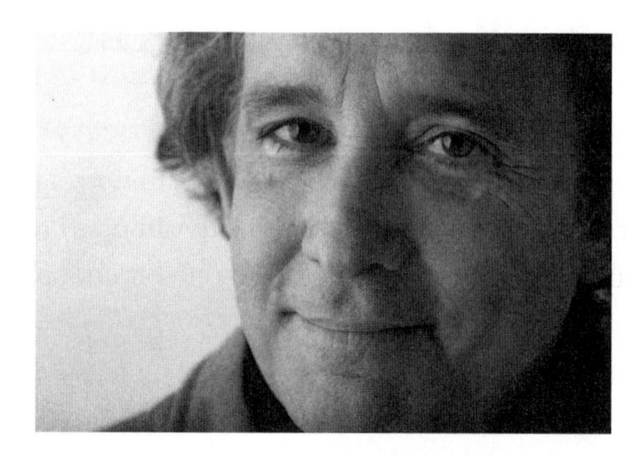

Andrew Harvey is an internationally acclaimed poet, novelist, translator, and spiritual teacher. He was born in South India in 1952, moved to England at age nine, and later attended Oxford University, where in 1973 he became a Fellow of All Souls College. In 1977, he returned to India for the first time since his childhood and underwent several mystical experiences, which began a series of initiations into different mystical traditions to learn their secrets and practices.

Harvey has taught at Oxford University, Cornell University, Hobart and William Smith Colleges, the California Institute of Integral Studies, and the University of Creation Spirituality (now Wisdom University), as well as at churches and spiritual centers throughout the United States, England, and Europe. He is the author of more than twenty-five books, including *Son of Man, The Direct Path, Hidden Journey, The Essential Mystics, The Way of Passion: A Celebration of Rumi, The Return of the Mother, A Journey in Ladakh, Sun at Midnight: A Memoir of the Dark Night,* and his most recent work, *The Hope: A Guide to Sacred Activism.*

Harvey was the subject of the 1993 BBC documentary *The Making of a Modern Mystic* and has appeared in several others, including *Rumi Turning Ecstatic, The Return of Rumi, The Consciousness of the Christ,* and a documentary on the life and work of Marion Woodman. His own 90-minute documentary *Sacred Activism* was produced by the Hartley Film Foundation in 2005. Several of his lectures are available on www.myss.com and on YouTube (see Web site below for contact information).

He is the founder and director of the Institute for Sacred Activism in Oak Park, Illinois, where he lives. His Web site is www.andrewharvey.net. He can be contacted at andrew@instituteforsacredactivism.org. He is available for interviews, lectures, courses, workshops, and one-on-one spiritual direction. For bookings, contact Jill Angelo at (928) 288-6097 and jill@institutefor sacredactivism.org.